METABOLIC CONFUSION DIET FOR ENDOMORPHS WOMEN

From Breakfast to Dinner, This Weight Loss Guide,
Healthy Eating Meal Plan & Tasty Recipes Provides an
optimal Balance Diet to Activate Your Metabolism,&
Achieve Your Fitness Goal.

Vince Cruise Sant

About The Book

Unlock Your Radiance: Embark on an Empowering Odyssey with 'Metabolic Confusion for Endomorph Women.' Elevate beyond diets, embrace holistic vitality, and rewrite your well-being story. From body wisdom to plateaus conquered, from delectable nutrient-rich recipes to the art of balanced living – this is your blueprint to radiant transformation. Your journey to a vibrant life begins now!

About The Author

Introducing Vince Cruise Sant, a seasoned nutritionist with over a decade of dedicated experience in transforming lives through the power of balanced nutrition. With an extensive background in the field, Vince has emerged as a respected figure, dedicated to guiding individuals toward achieving their health and wellness aspirations.

With a wealth of practical knowledge and a deep understanding of nutrition and metabolism, Vince's expertise extends beyond theory. Having positively impacted the lives of more than 300 individuals, he stands as a testament to the tangible results his guidance brings.

Vince's approach transcends the conventional, recognizing the individuality of each person's journey toward well-being. His methodology seamlessly blends scientific insights with real-world application, ensuring that his advice is not only attainable but also sustainable.

Recognized as a trusted advisor and advocate for balanced nutrition, Vince Cruise Sant's commitment to empowering individuals is unwavering. His reputation as a compassionate and knowledgeable guide underscores his dedication to helping others unlock their full potential.

Whether you're a newcomer to the path of wellness or seeking to refine your existing practices, Vince's expertise will inspire and educate. Prepare to embark on a transformative journey led by a visionary who firmly believes that vibrant health is an achievable reality. With Vince's guidance, your pursuit of lasting well-being is poised for exceptional success.

TABLE OF CONTENTS

INTRODUCTION

"Metabolic Confusion" is a concept that has gained popularity in recent years as a unique approach to weight management and overall metabolic health. It involves strategically introducing variations in both your dietary and exercise routines to prevent your body from adapting to a specific regimen.

At its core, metabolic confusion aims to prevent the body from settling into a routine that could lead to stagnation in terms of weight loss or muscle growth. The basic idea is that by keeping your body guessing and avoiding a consistent pattern, you can potentially stimulate your metabolism and achieve more consistent progress over time.

Metabolic confusion can be applied in different ways:

Dietary Variation: This involves altering your macronutrient intake and caloric levels at different intervals. For instance, you might have days of higher carbohydrate intake followed by days of lower intake. This variance is believed to keep your metabolism active and adaptable.

Caloric Cycling: Similar to varying macronutrients, this approach involves changing your overall caloric intake. Some days you might consume more calories, while on others you consume fewer. This fluctuation is thought to prevent your body from adjusting to a fixed calorie count.

Intermittent Fasting: Incorporating intermittent fasting patterns is another facet of metabolic confusion. Adjusting the timing of your meals and fasting periods can impact how your body processes energy and manages fat.

Exercise Diversity: Metabolic confusion extends to your workout routine. Instead of sticking to the same exercises and intensity levels, you'd incorporate various types of workouts, such as high-intensity interval training (HIIT), strength training, and cardio.

Timing and Frequency Tweaks: Altering the timing and frequency of meals and workouts is also part of metabolic confusion. Changing the time you work out or adjusting meal frequency adds an element of unpredictability to your routine.

It's worth noting that while metabolic confusion presents an intriguing approach, it's not a one-size-fits-all solution.

Metabolic confusion might particularly appeal to those who've hit a plateau in their weight loss journey or those seeking to revitalize their fitness progress. However, like any lifestyle change, it should be tailored to your individual needs and preferences.

Benefits of Metabolic Confusion

Metabolic confusion has various potential benefits, which have contributed to its appeal as a method of weight loss and fitness. Here's a rundown of some of the main advantages:

1. Plateau Prevention:

Metabolic confusion makes it difficult for the body to adjust to a new diet or exercise plan.

By avoiding adaptation, you may be able to escape weight loss or muscle-building plateaus that are frequent with continuous regimens.

2. Higher Metabolic Flexibility:

The method helps the body to become metabolically flexible, which means it can switch between using carbs and fats for energy effectively.

10

This adaptability has the potential to improve fat-burning and overall energy consumption.

3. Constant Calorie Burn:

Dietary and exercise regimen variety might help maintain the metabolism active.

This may result in a constant calorie expenditure throughout the day, even when resting.

4. Increased Fat Loss:

By preventing the body from adjusting to a given calorie intake or macronutrient distribution, metabolic confusion may stimulate fat loss.

Because of the continually shifting environment, the body may rely more on stored fat for energy.

5. Muscle Retention:

Changing up your workouts and intensity levels might assist you in avoiding muscular adaption and breakdown.

This is especially crucial while trying to lose weight since preserving muscle mass promotes a faster metabolic rate.

6. Improved Fitness Progress: The method can lead to gains in strength, endurance, and general fitness.

Workouts that are varied test multiple muscular groups and energy systems, which contributes to overall fitness improvement.

7. Psychological Participation:

Metabolic confusion keeps your routine fresh and intriguing.

Trying new workouts, changing up your diet, and embracing change might help you avoid boredom and stay motivated.

8. Adaptable to Personal Preferences:

Metabolic confusion may be tailored to various food habits and fitness levels.

It is adaptable and may be tailored to the needs of each individual.

9. Potential Hormonal Advantages:

Cycling between caloric deficit and maintenance phases might help to avoid hormonal abnormalities that can arise with continuous calorie restriction.

This may aid in the maintenance of balanced hormone levels, which are essential for general well-being.

10. Long-term viability:

The method supports a way of living that avoids rigid and boring routines.

This can lead to a long-term, sustainable method of eating and exercise.

11. Overcoming Weight Loss Stagnation:

Metabolic confusion is especially beneficial for people who have reached weight reduction plateaus since it provides fresh factors to re-start progress.

12. Individualized Approach:

Individual objectives, interests, and lifestyles may all be accommodated via metabolic confusion.

Personalization increases the chances of success and long-term adherence.

Tailoring the Metabolic Confusion Approach for Endomorph Women

Tailoring the Metabolic Confusion approach for endomorph women means adjusting the strategy to fit their specific needs. Endomorphs are more likely to have a bit more body fat and a slower metabolism, which can make managing weight a bit trickier. Here's how to make the Metabolic Confusion approach work well for endomorph women:

1. Choose Healthy Foods: Focus on eating foods that are good for you and packed with nutrients.

Pick foods that have complex carbs, lean proteins, and healthy fats.

2. Change How Much You Eat: Keep an eye on how many calories you're eating, especially since endomorphs can gain weight more easily.

Switch between eating more and eating less to keep your body guessing.

3. Mix Up Your Nutrients: Rotate the amount of carbs, proteins, and fats you eat, but remember to get enough protein.

Some days eat more carbs, and some days eat fewer, so your body doesn't get used to a specific pattern.

4. Get Stronger: Do strength training exercises regularly to build and keep your muscles strong.

Muscles help boost your metabolism and give you a more toned look.

5. Try Different Workouts: Do both steady and intense workouts, like quick bursts of intense exercise.

Intense workouts can help you burn calories even after you're done exercising.

6. Think About When You Eat: Intermittent fasting might be a good idea, but make sure it fits your needs.

Eat during certain times and fast during others, but still make sure to get the nutrients you need.

7. Watch Your Carbs: Be careful with carbs, especially sugary and simple ones.

Choose whole grains, vegetables, and fruits for lasting energy.

8. Eat Enough Protein: Protein helps your muscles grow and repair, which is extra important for endomorphs.

Have lean protein with each meal to feel full and keep your muscles healthy.

9. Pay Attention to Portions: Since endomorphs tend to store extra fat, keep your portion sizes in check.

Make sure you're not eating too much, even if the food is healthy.

10. Be Patient and Keep Going: Sticking to your plan and being consistent is super important, even if you don't see big changes right away.

It might take a bit longer for endomorphs to see results, so don't give up!

11. Drink Water and Sleep: Stay hydrated and get enough sleep to help your metabolism and overall health.

12. Listen to Your Body: Pay attention to how your body reacts to different foods and exercises.

Change your approach based on how you feel and what's working for you.

13. Get Expert Help: Consider talking to a dietitian or fitness expert who knows about endomorphs.

They can give you advice that fits your body's needs.

How This Book Will Guide You

This book is a thorough guide to understanding, implementing, and succeeding with the metabolic confusion technique designed exclusively for endomorph women. Here's how the book can help you along the way:

Understanding Metabolic Confusion: The book begins by defining metabolic confusion, its advantages, and how it may be tailored to endomorph women. This lays the groundwork for your future studies.

Endomorph Body Types: You'll obtain a thorough grasp of endomorph body types, including their traits and problems. This understanding enables you to identify your specific requirements.

The Science of Metabolic Confusion: You'll learn about metabolism and why the metabolic confusion technique works for endomorphs. This understanding provides you with the "why" behind the technique.

The Metabolic Confusion Diet ideas: This chapter describes the approach's key ideas, such as macronutrient cycling and calorie fluctuation. You'll discover how to apply these concepts to your eating habits.

Making Your Metabolic Confusion Meal Plan: The book walks you through the process of creating a customized meal plan that adheres to metabolic confusion concepts. Sample meal plans tailored to various calorie requirements will help you get started.

Implementing Metabolic Confusion exercises: You'll learn how to plan your exercises so that you get the most out of the metabolic confusion effect. The chapter discusses how to incorporate strength training, HIIT, and other activities into your routine to keep your body responsive.

Overcoming Obstacles and Maintaining Consistency: This chapter discusses frequent roadblocks like as cravings and emotional eating. There are various ways to keep consistency in social contexts. This advice keeps you on track in real-world settings.

Meal Prep and Recipes for Success: Practical meal prep guidance and a variety of nutritious recipes save you time and help you achieve your nutritional objectives.

Meal planning is made easier with grocery shopping and cooking skills tips.

Listening to Your Body: Plateaus and Adjustments: Learn to read your body's messages and make the appropriate modifications. Breaking through plateaus strategies guarantee that your development remains consistent.

Beyond the Diet: This chapter highlights the need for a holistic approach, which includes stress management, sleep, and a positive mentality. You'll be prepared to make long-term adjustments.

CHAPTER 1

DEMYSTIFYING ENDOMORPH BODY TYPES

Exploring Different Body Types

There are three primary body types, often referred to as somatotypes, which describe general physical characteristics and tendencies related to metabolism and body composition. These body types are ectomorph, mesomorph, and endomorph. Each body type has distinct features and traits. Here's a comprehensive explanation of each:

1. Ectomorph:

Ectomorphs are often characterized by their lean and slender physical appearance. They possess certain distinctive traits that contribute to their unique body composition and metabolism.

Body Characteristics: Ectomorphs typically have a narrow bone structure, which is reflected in their slim wrists, ankles, and shoulders. They often have a delicate, elongated build with relatively little body fat.

Metabolism and Weight Management: Ectomorphs tend to have a fast metabolism, meaning their bodies burn calories efficiently. This characteristic makes it challenging for them to gain weight, including muscle mass. Ectomorphs may find it difficult to put on muscle despite their efforts to increase calorie intake.

Muscle Development: While ectomorphs might struggle to gain muscle, their body type often enables them to maintain a lean and defined appearance even with modest exercise. However, building significant muscle mass might require consistent strength training and higher caloric intake.

2. Mesomorph:

Mesomorphs are known for their naturally athletic and muscular physique. They possess traits that make them well-suited for physical activities and muscle development.

Body Characteristics: Mesomorphs generally have a well-proportioned body with a balanced bone structure. They often exhibit a naturally athletic appearance with broad shoulders, a narrow waist, and a noticeable muscle definition.

Muscle and Strength: One of the key features of mesomorphs is their ability to gain muscle mass relatively easily. Their bodies respond well to strength training and tend to show visible muscle definition even without extensive exercise.

Metabolism and Weight Management: Mesomorphs tend to have a moderate metabolism, allowing them to manage their weight more easily than endomorphs. They can both gain muscle and lose fat with appropriate dietary and exercise strategies.

3. Endomorph:

Endomorphs typically have a softer and rounder physique. They exhibit certain characteristics that influence their body composition and how they respond to diet and exercise.

Body Characteristics: Endomorphs often have a wider bone structure and a rounder overall appearance. They might have a fuller face and a higher percentage of body fat compared to ectomorphs and mesomorphs.

Metabolism and Weight Management: Endomorphs usually have a slower metabolism, which can make it more challenging for them to lose weight and maintain a lean physique. They tend to store fat more easily, especially around the abdomen, hips, and thighs.

Fat Storage and Muscle Building: While endomorphs might find it easier to gain both muscle and fat, it's important for them to carefully manage their caloric intake and choose appropriate exercise routines to strike a balance between muscle development and fat loss.

Characteristics of Endomorph Women: Challenges and Strengths

Endomorph women have specific physical and metabolic characteristics that influence their body composition, response to diet and exercise, and overall health. Here's a breakdown of the characteristics, challenges, and strengths commonly associated with endomorph body types:

Characteristics of Endomorph Women:

Body Shape and Composition: Endomorph women typically exhibit a soft and curvy body shape. They often have a rounder appearance with a wider waist, fuller hips, and a generous amount of body fat.

Fat Distribution: A hallmark trait of endomorphs is their tendency to store fat more easily. This fat accumulation primarily occurs around the lower abdomen, hips, and thighs, contributing to their characteristic curves.

Muscle Definition: Due to a higher body fat percentage, muscle definition may be less pronounced in endomorph women compared to other body types. Muscles might be less visible under the layer of stored fat.

Bone Structure: Endomorphs often possess a sturdy bone structure with broader shoulders and hips. This robust frame adds to their more solid appearance.

Weight Management Challenges: Managing weight can pose challenges for endomorph women due to their slower metabolic rate and predisposition to store fat. Weight loss might require more effort compared to other body types.

Challenges Faced by Endomorph Women:

Weight Control and Fat Loss: One of the main challenges is the struggle to control weight, especially fat. The body's inclination to store fat can make losing excess weight a more complex endeavor.

Fat Loss Difficulty: Endomorphs often find it harder to shed body fat and achieve a lean physique. Their bodies tend to hold onto fat reserves, making fat loss efforts more demanding.

Balancing Muscle Gain: While endomorphs can build muscle effectively, increasing muscle mass might also lead to some fat gain due to the body's propensity to store energy.

Metabolic Rate: The slower metabolic rate of endomorphs can be a hurdle in weight management. It means they burn calories at a reduced rate, potentially making weight loss more challenging.

Strengths Exhibited by Endomorph Women:

Muscle Potential: Despite the challenges, endomorph women possess an advantage in terms of muscle development. Their bodies respond well to resistance training, allowing them to build strong and well-defined muscles.

Strength and Power: The solid bone structure and greater muscle potential of endomorphs can result in impressive strength and power. They often excel in activities requiring physical strength, such as weightlifting or certain sports.

Satiety and Appetite Control: The combination of muscle mass potential and higher body fat can lead to enhanced feelings of fullness after meals. This can contribute to better appetite control.

Fitness Progress: With consistent effort, endomorphs can achieve remarkable fitness progress. Their bodies adapt well to strength training, leading to noticeable improvements in muscle definition and overall fitness.

Energy Resilience: The body's tendency to store fat can provide a source of energy reserves. This attribute can be advantageous in situations where food availability is limited.

The Role of Genetics in Body Composition and Weight Management

Genetics plays a substantial role in shaping an individual's body composition and how their body interacts with efforts to manage weight. Here's a more detailed exploration of the impact of genetics in these areas:

1. Body Composition:

Genetic factors wield influence over several aspects of body composition, encompassing:

- Distribution of Body Fat: Genetics contributes significantly to where the body tends to store fat. Some people naturally accumulate fat around the abdomen (the "apple" shape), while others deposit it in the hips and thighs (the "pear" shape).

- Potential for Muscle Mass: Genetic predisposition also affects how readily someone can build and maintain muscle mass. Certain individuals are genetically inclined toward muscle development.

- Metabolic Rate: Your basal metabolic rate (BMR), the rate at which your body burns calories at rest, bears a genetic element. Certain individuals possess a naturally higher BMR, resulting in more calories burned even during periods of inactivity.

- Body Typing: Genetic factors contribute to the definition of body types like ectomorphs, mesomorphs, and endomorphs. This classification affects natural physique, predisposition to muscle gain or fat storage, and overall metabolic tendencies.

2. Weight Management:

Genetics also shape how your body reacts to attempts at weight management:

- Weight Set Point: Genetics may dictate a preferred weight range for your body, often referred to as the weight set point. Your body may resist straying from this range, complicating efforts to maintain significant weight changes.
- Appetite Regulation: Genetic factors influence how the body regulates hunger and fullness. Some individuals might experience more robust hunger signals, making the control of food intake more challenging.
- Fat Storage and Hormones: Genetic variations impact the body's responses to hormones that govern appetite and fat storage, such as insulin and leptin.
- Dietary Response: Genetics can lead to varied reactions to different diets based on one's genetic makeup. For instance, certain individuals might experience more effective weight loss on a low-carb diet compared to a balanced one.
- Exercise Impact: Genetics also play a role in determining how the body reacts to exercise. Certain individuals might observe more rapid muscle growth or

fat loss when engaging in specific types of exercise due to their genetic inclinations.

3. Interaction Between Genetics and Environment:

It's important to recognize that genetics and environment interact, including elements like diet, physical activity, and lifestyle choices:

- Gene Expression: While genetic makeup remains fixed, lifestyle choices can influence how specific genes are expressed. This fascinating field is known as epigenetics.
- Adaptation to Environment: The body adjusts to its environment. For instance, while genetics may predispose you to store fat, adopting a healthy lifestyle can help mitigate this tendency.

4. Tailoring Strategies to Individuals:

Comprehending your genetic inclinations can guide customized approaches to weight management. Although genetics undoubtedly play a role, lifestyle factors such as diet, exercise, sleep, and stress management are under your control and can significantly impact your health and weight.

Genetics wield considerable influence over body composition, weight management, and how the body responds to different interventions. While genetic makeup remains unchangeable, making informed decisions can optimize your health and well-being. Collaborating with healthcare professionals or registered dietitians can aid in devising a tailored approach that takes your genetics and personal needs into account.

CHAPTER 2

THE SCIENCE BEHIND METABOLIC CONFUSION

Metabolism Unveiled: How Your Body Burns Calories

The process of burning calories, also known as energy expenditure, is a complex and continuous physiological process that occurs within the human body. Here's a breakdown of how your body burns calories:

1. Basal Metabolic Rate (BMR):

Think of your body as a busy factory that never stops working, even when you're asleep or just sitting quietly. This factory, your body, needs energy to keep all its machines running smoothly. We call this energy the Basal Metabolic Rate (BMR). It's the energy your body uses to do essential tasks like breathing, keeping your heart beating, making new cells, and maintaining a comfortable temperature. This energy is measured in calories. Factors like your age, gender, weight, height, and even your genes determine how many calories your body needs just to stay alive and functioning.

2. Physical Activity:

Imagine every movement you make as another opportunity for your body to burn calories. When you walk, run, play sports, or even dance around your room, you're using up energy. This is called physical activity, and it comes in three forms:

- Non-Exercise Activity Thermogenesis (NEAT): This is a fancy term for the energy you use when you're not exercising but doing regular things like walking to the store, standing up, or tapping your foot.
- Exercise Activity: These are the planned activities where you intentionally move your body, like going for a bike ride, doing yoga, or lifting weights at the gym. The harder and longer you move, the more calories you burn.
- Thermic Effect of Food (TEF): Eating isn't just about enjoying delicious meals. Your body spends energy to digest and process the food you eat. This energy usage is known as the Thermic Effect of Food (TEF). Some foods, like protein-rich foods, make your body work harder to process, using up more energy in the process.

3. Adaptive Thermogenesis:

Imagine you're out in the cold, and your body starts shivering to keep warm. This shivering is like your body's way of burning extra calories to create heat. This process is called adaptive thermogenesis, where your body adapts to changes in temperature or situations by using up more energy.

4. Hormonal Regulation:

Inside your body, there are tiny messengers called hormones. These hormones help control how your body uses energy. For instance, thyroid hormones act like traffic signals, telling your body how fast to burn calories. When you're stressed or excited, adrenaline is released, which speeds up your calorie burning, especially if you're doing something active.

5. Muscle Mass:

Think of your muscles as little calorie-burning engines. The more muscle you have, the more energy your body needs to keep those engines running. This means that having more muscle mass can help you burn more calories even when you're not moving much.

6. Genetic Factors:

Just like you inherit traits like eye color from your parents, your genes also influence how your body burns calories. Some lucky folks have genes that give them a higher BMR, making their bodies burn calories faster. Others might have genes that make them naturally inclined to be more active.

In a nutshell, your body is a remarkable energy-burning machine. Whether you're catching Z's, going for a jog, or simply enjoying a meal, you're using up calories in various ways. By understanding how these processes work and making informed choices about food, movement, and lifestyle, you can harness the power of calorie burning to maintain good health and achieve your wellness goals.

How Does Metabolic Confusion Works

Metabolic confusion refers to a food and exercise approach that aims to maintain the responsiveness and adaptability of one's metabolism. The approach entails manipulating one's calorie intake, distribution of macronutrients, and intensity of physical activity to hinder the body's adaptation to a certain regimen. The objective of this technique is to maximize the reduction of body fat, increase muscle mass, and enhance overall metabolic efficiency. Metabolic confusion operates in the following manner:

1. Caloric Fluctuation: The concept of metabolic confusion entails the periodic alteration of one's calorie consumption. Caloric intake fluctuates on different days, with some days exhibiting higher consumption and others demonstrating lower consumption. This phenomenon hinders the body's ability to adapt to a stable caloric intake, hence resulting in a stationary metabolic rate. The diversification of calorie consumption serves to enhance metabolic activity and promote adipose tissue reduction by averting the deceleration of metabolic rate resulting from extended caloric restriction.

2. Macronutrient Cycling: In conjunction with caloric fluctuation, metabolic confusion includes the manipulation of macronutrient allocation (carbohydrates, proteins, and fats) within one's dietary regimen. On certain occasions, individuals may want to enhance their carbohydrate consumption, whilst on other occasions, they may choose to augment their protein intake. This practice prevents the body from developing proficiency in metabolizing a certain nutrient, hence enhancing the efficiency of nutrient use.

3. Intermittent Fasting or Meal time: The concept of metabolic confusion encompasses the utilization of intermittent fasting or the manipulation of meal time. Intermittent fasting is a dietary approach characterized by alternating periods of eating and fasting. This particular pattern can generate fluctuations in calorie expenditure and influence insulin sensitivity, which may potentially augment the process of fat reduction and improve metabolic adaptability.

4. Variability in Exercise: The exercise component of metabolic confusion emphasizes the manipulation of intensity, duration, and modality of physical activities. Various types of exercise, such as High-Intensity Interval Training (HIIT), strength training, and cardiovascular activities, are alternated. This phenomenon hinders the body's ability to acclimate to a particular training regimen, resulting in enhanced reduction of adipose tissue, augmentation of muscular development, and improvement of cardiovascular endurance.

5. Mitigating Plateau Phenomenon: A fundamental objective of metabolic confusion is to circumvent the occurrence of weight loss plateaus. When an individual's body becomes acclimated to a specific routine, it develops increased efficiency in energy conservation, perhaps resulting in a plateau in progress. By regularly altering factors such as calorie intake and exercise, individuals may effectively stimulate their bodies to consistently adapt, avoiding performance plateaus and maintaining an active metabolism.

6. Hormonal Response: The perturbation of metabolism can also exert an influence on the hormonal milieu associated with metabolic processes, including insulin, leptin, and thyroid hormones. Hormonal oscillations have a crucial role in the regulation of hunger, fat storage, and energy expenditure, hence facilitating weight reduction and enhancing body composition.

7. Consistency and a Long-Term method: Although the phrase "metabolic confusion" may appear extreme, this method emphasizes maintaining a healthy and balanced diet, as well as engaging in regular exercise. The importance of consistency cannot be overstated, as the technique in question is specifically formulated to yield enduring outcomes, prioritizing long-term sustainability over immediate, transient alterations.

8. Variability among Individuals: It is crucial to acknowledge that there might be variations in individual reactions to metabolic confusion. Various factors, such as genetic predisposition, advancing age, gender, and pre-existing health issues, might exert an impact on the physiological response of the body to this particular technique. Therefore, it is advisable to customize the plan according to individual requirements and seek guidance from a healthcare practitioner before implementing substantial modifications to one's dietary and physical activity regimen.

Hormones and Metabolic Rate: Understanding the Connection

1. Thyroid Hormones: Imagine your thyroid gland as the control center for your metabolism. It produces hormones called thyroxine (T4) and triiodothyronine (T3). These hormones are like the gas pedal that sets the pace of your metabolic engine. They influence important functions such as how fast your heart beats, your body temperature, and most importantly, how efficiently your cells use energy. When levels of these hormones are low (hypothyroidism), your metabolic engine slows down, potentially leading to weight gain and sluggishness. On the flip side, when these hormone levels are high (hyperthyroidism), your metabolic engine revs up, potentially causing weight loss and increased energy.

2. Insulin:

Think of insulin as the key that unlocks your cells, allowing them to use glucose (sugar) from your bloodstream for energy or storage. It's produced by your pancreas and is a key player in metabolism. When you eat, your body releases insulin to help your cells absorb glucose. If you become resistant to insulin, which can happen with poor lifestyle habits, your cells don't respond as effectively. This can lead to elevated blood sugar levels and a decrease in metabolic efficiency.

3. Leptin:

Picture leptin as your body's satiety messenger. It's released by your fat cells and signals to your brain that you're full. This hormone is like a traffic light that says, "Stop eating, you're satisfied!" Leptin is important for regulating your body weight and metabolism. However, when your brain becomes resistant to leptin's signals, you might feel hungrier and struggle to maintain a healthy weight.

4. Ghrelin:

Meet ghrelin, the hormone responsible for your tummy's grumbling. Ghrelin is produced in your stomach and is your body's way of saying, "Hey, it's time to eat!" Before meals, ghrelin levels rise, prompting you to seek out food. It's like your body's hunger alarm. This hormone also influences how your body uses energy, impacting your metabolic rate.

5. Cortisol:

Think of cortisol as your body's stress responder. It's released by your adrenal glands during stressful situations. While it helps manage stress, chronically elevated cortisol levels can lead to some not-so-great outcomes. Picture cortisol as a messenger that tells your body to store fat, especially around your midsection. This can influence how your body uses energy and affects your overall body composition.

6. Growth Hormone:

Imagine growth hormone (GH) as your body's repair and renewal crew. It's produced by your pituitary gland and plays a big role in muscle growth, metabolism, and more. GH helps break down fats for energy and encourages your body to use fats as fuel. This has a direct impact on your metabolic rate and how your body uses energy.

7. Sex Hormones (Estrogen and Testosterone):

Picture sex hormones as the sculptors of your body's composition. Estrogen in women and testosterone in men play crucial roles in shaping how your body stores fat, builds muscle and grows. As these hormones fluctuate, such as during menopause or andropause, they can influence your metabolic rate and how your body processes energy.

8. Metabolic Rate and Age:

Imagine your hormones as the orchestrators of a symphony. As you age, this symphony changes, and hormonal shifts occur. Sex hormone production decreases in both men and women, affecting muscle mass, fat distribution, and overall metabolism. This symphony's changes can influence how efficiently your metabolic engine runs.

CHAPTER 3

PRINCIPLES OF THE METABOLIC CONFUSION DIET

Cycling Macronutrients

Let us go into the notion of cycling macronutrients, namely carbs, proteins, and fats, in a more scholarly manner.

Optimizing Nutrition by Cycling Macronutrients

Consider conceptualizing the human body as a meticulously calibrated apparatus necessitating a harmonious amalgamation of several energy sources to optimize its performance. The fuel source is comprised of three primary macronutrients, namely carbs, proteins, and lipids. The practice of macronutrient cycling is purposefully altering the quantities and ratios of these essential nutrients in one's dietary intake throughout certain periods. This strategy provides a multitude of advantages that add to one's overall health and fitness endeavors.

Carbohydrates as the Primary Source of Energy

Carbohydrates may be conceptualized as the principal source of energy that drives the physiological processes within the human body. They supply the necessary energy for daily tasks, ranging from basic locomotion to more vigorous physical exertion. Carbohydrates may be likened to rapidly combusting logs in a fire, as they provide an immediate surge of energy. The practice of manipulating carbohydrate consumption following one's degree of physical activity is referred to as carbohydrate cycling. During periods of heightened physical activity or participation in intense exercise regimens, it may be necessary to augment one's carbohydrate consumption to restore depleted glycogen reserves and meet the increased energy demands imposed on the body.

Proteins: Fundamental Units of Muscular Development

Proteins serve as fundamental constituents responsible for the repair and maintenance of bodily structures. Consider them as the laborers involved in the process of refurbishing the physical structure that is your corporeal form. The practice of regulating protein consumption in the context of cycling entails the deliberate effort to get a sufficient quantity of this essential nutrient to facilitate the process of muscle recovery and development. During periods characterized by heightened levels of physical activity or strength training, it may be advisable to marginally increase one's protein consumption to provide the necessary building blocks for muscle recovery and growth.

Fats: Sustained Energy and Vital Functions

Fats might be conceptualized as the slow-burning logs within a fire, offering a protracted release of energy over an extended duration. They play a crucial role in several physiological processes, such as the synthesis of hormones and the assimilation of vitamins that are soluble in fat. The concept of cycling fats involves the consumption of nutritious sources of fats in appropriate and well-proportioned quantities. Although fats may not serve as the major source of immediate energy, they are essential for sustaining general health and can be particularly advantageous during periods of lower-intensity activity or restorative processes.

The Advantages of Cycling:

- Improved Performance: By modifying one's macronutrient consumption following their degree of physical activity, individuals may supply their bodies with the appropriate quantity and quality of energy required. This phenomenon has the potential to enhance exercise performance and boost levels of energy.

- The strategic manipulation of carbohydrate intake, known as carbohydrate cycling, is an effective approach for both maximizing fat reduction and maintaining lean muscle composition. Sufficient consumption of protein facilitates the development and maintenance of muscular tissue, while the inclusion of nutritious fats in one's diet plays a role in maintaining a harmonious hormonal equilibrium.

- Metabolic flexibility refers to the ability of an individual's metabolism to adapt and adjust in response to changes in macronutrient ratios. Regularly altering these ratios is believed to promote metabolic adaptability. This phenomenon hinders the body's ability to optimize the digestion of a particular nutrient, perhaps resulting in the occurrence of plateaus.

- The optimization of nutrients: The practice of cycling macronutrients facilitates the achievement of a comprehensive intake of vital nutrients. Every macronutrient has distinct advantages, and by including cycling in your diet, you can guarantee that your body receives a comprehensive range of essential nutrients.

Caloric Variation: The Key to Preventing Plateaus

Caloric variation stands as a strategic method aimed at circumventing plateaus encountered in the pursuit of health and fitness objectives. It entails purposefully altering one's daily caloric intake systematically, thus thwarting the propensity of the body to adapt to a consistent caloric regimen. This deliberate fluctuation of caloric consumption serves to rejuvenate metabolic processes, optimize adipose tissue reduction, and amplify overall outcomes. Let us delve into the intricacies of how caloric variation operates:

Deconstructing Caloric Variation:

In envisioning the body as a pliable organism, it becomes evident that maintaining a persistent caloric equilibrium

47

over time can prompt metabolic homeostasis. This equilibrium often precipitates a plateau—a juncture where weight loss or muscle gain subsides or halts entirely. Caloric variation assumes a pivotal role within this context.

1. Adaption Evasion: Caloric variation pertains to the cyclic adjustment of one's daily caloric intake. The oscillation between periods of elevated caloric consumption and instances of restrained caloric intake functions as a stratagem to obviate habituation. The inherent unpredictability of energy availability mitigates the inclination toward metabolic adaptation.

2. Augmenting Metabolic Activity: Metabolic processes mirror a controlled fire. A continuous supply of identical fuel (calories) may provoke a slowdown akin to the dwindling flames. Conversely, infusing intermittent increments or intensities into the fire augments its vigor. Similarly, caloric variation invigorates metabolic dynamics, preempting complacency.

3. Overcoming Stagnation: Akin to an expedition interspersed with halts for respite, the journey towards fitness aspirations requires occasional deviations. Caloric variation mirrors these halts, ensuring that one's path is not characterized by monotonous linearity.

4. Individualization and Sustainability:

Caloric variation transpires in the context of individualization. The strategy necessitates meticulous calibration to accommodate distinct aims, activity levels, and predilections. The intention is not radical caloric deprivation on low days or excessive indulgence on high days, but rather the orchestrated fluctuation that engenders a constructive adaptive response. The sustained nature of this approach is paramount.

5. Optimizing Lipolysis and Myogenesis: Caloric variation engenders a favorable metabolic milieu conducive to accentuated lipid mobilization for energy expenditure. This underpins expedited adipose tissue reduction. Furthermore, the strategy safeguards muscle preservation and growth, as higher caloric days provide the requisite energy for strenuous workouts and the ensuing recovery process.

6. Hormonal Equilibrium: Caloric variation contributes to the harmonization of hormonal equilibrium, particularly about hormones such as leptin and thyroid hormones.

These regulatory agents play pivotal roles in mediating metabolic processes and satiety responses. The avoidance of protracted caloric restriction safeguards against hormonal imbalances that might otherwise impede progress.

Intermittent Fasting and its Synergy with Metabolic Confusion

Intermittent fasting (IF) and metabolic confusion represent distinct yet complementary approaches to achieving optimal metabolic health and overall well-being. Intermittent fasting involves cycling between periods of eating and fasting, while metabolic confusion centers around varying dietary and exercise parameters. Understanding their synergy can provide insights into how these strategies can collectively enhance metabolic flexibility and promote positive physiological outcomes.

Intermittent Fasting: Quick Recap

Intermittent fasting is like a pattern of eating that involves cycles of eating and not eating. It's kind of like having scheduled meal and snack times and then giving your body a break from food. This can help your body burn stored fat for energy and do some repairs inside your cells.

Metabolic Confusion: A Concise Understanding:

Metabolic confusion is about keeping your body guessing. Instead of sticking to the same routine, you mix things up. Sometimes you eat more calories, sometimes fewer. You change the types of foods you eat and switch up your exercise routines. This prevents your body from getting too comfortable and helps you burn fat and build muscle better.

How They Team Up:

- *Using Fat for Energy:* Intermittent fasting makes your body use its fat stores for energy during fasting times. When you also experience metabolic confusion, your body gets even better at using those fat stores. This teamwork helps you lose weight more effectively.
- *Helping Insulin and Hormones:* Both intermittent fasting and metabolic confusion can make your body listen better to insulin, which is good for controlling your blood sugar. They also work together to balance other hormones that help with your metabolism.

- *Being Flexible with Metabolism:* Imagine your body can switch between using different types of energy, like switching between gas and electricity for a car. Intermittent fasting helps your body learn to use different types of energy sources. Metabolic confusion makes sure your body keeps switching between these sources. This combo helps you manage your weight better.
- *Avoiding Stuck Points:* Sometimes our bodies get used to the same routine and stop changing. This is called hitting a plateau. When you use both intermittent fasting and metabolic confusion, your body keeps changing and doesn't get stuck. This helps you keep making progress on your fitness journey.
- *Cleaning Up and Repairing:* Intermittent fasting can help your cells clean up and repair themselves. When you add metabolic confusion, your cells get different nutrients at different times, which helps them fix and maintain themselves even better.

Important Points:

Remember, even though these two strategies work well together, everyone is different. What works for one person might not work the same for another. It's a good idea to talk to experts like doctors or dietitians before making big changes to your eating and exercise routine.

Intermittent fasting and metabolic confusion are like a dynamic duo for your body's metabolism. They team up to help you burn fat, control hormones, stay flexible with energy, avoid plateaus, and even do some cellular tidying up. Using these strategies together can give you a powerful boost on your path to better health and fitness.

CHAPTER 4

CRAFTING YOUR METABOLIC CONFUSION MEAL PLAN

Designing a Balanced Diet for Endomorphs: Nutrient Ratios

Designing a nutritionally balanced regimen for individuals classified as endomorphs entails meticulous consideration of nutrient ratios conducive to their distinct metabolic and physiological characteristics. Given their predisposition to heightened fat storage, the formulation of nutrient distribution assumes paramount importance, aiming to facilitate fat reduction, safeguard lean muscle mass, and foster holistic well-being. The following discourse elucidates the fundamental nutrient ratios integral to formulating a judicious diet for endomorphs:

1. Protein Intake: Sustaining Lean Muscle

Endomorphs' dietary regimen should underscore the prominence of protein intake, crucial for the preservation of lean muscle mass during the pursuit of fat loss objectives. A protein content comprising approximately 25-30% of total daily caloric intake serves as an initial benchmark. Optimal sources encompass lean proteins such as poultry, fish, lean meats, eggs, legumes, and plant-based alternatives.

2. Carbohydrates: Provision of Metabolic Substrates

A judicious carbohydrate allocation of approximately 40-45% of daily caloric intake is recommended. The selection of complex carbohydrates—predominantly derived from whole grains, fruits, vegetables, and legumes—is advised. This choice augments sustained energy provision and the inclusion of dietary fiber, pivotal for satiety regulation and digestive health.

3. Dietary Fats: Essential Lipids for Metabolic Equilibrium

Fats should comprise approximately 25-30% of daily caloric intake. Emphasis should be placed on sourcing healthy fats from avocados, nuts, seeds, olive oil, and omega-3-rich fatty fish. These lipid constituents are integral to hormone synthesis, energy production, and holistic physiological functioning.

4. Fiber: Facilitating Satiety and Metabolic Efficiency

The inclusion of dietary fiber assumes paramount significance for endomorphs. Ample incorporation of whole grains, fruits, vegetables, legumes, and nuts provides the requisite fiber content, instrumental in fostering satiety, managing caloric intake, and optimizing digestive processes.

5. Micronutrients: Foundation of Metabolic Homeostasis

Micronutrients in the form of vitamins and minerals play pivotal roles in modulating metabolic pathways, energy generation, and overall homeostasis. A diverse assortment of colorful fruits and vegetables should be emphasized to encompass a broad spectrum of essential micronutrients. Supplemental interventions should be undertaken judiciously, preferably under professional guidance.

6. Hydration: The Hydromineral Nexus

Hydration, an often underestimated facet, is integral to a balanced dietary paradigm. Hydration maintains metabolic efficiency, aids in digestion, and sustains physiological equilibrium. The adoption of adequate hydration practices is thus imperative.

7. Portion Regulation: Caloric Equilibrium and Body Composition

Vigilance over portion sizes stands pivotal to caloric control, a tenet fundamental to weight management. While nutrient ratios are central, caloric magnitude remains a cardinal determinant. Mindful portion regulation and vigilant caloric accounting are efficacious measures.

8. Temporal Nutrient Distribution: Chronobiological Influences

Temporal nutrient distribution is germane to maintaining metabolic stability. Dispersing meals and snacks across the day curbs fluctuations in blood glucose levels mitigates hunger pangs, and provides sustained energy reservoirs. Ensuring protein sufficiency across meals fosters muscle retention.

9. Individual Variability: Cognizance of Heterogeneity

Heterogeneity characterizes individual responses to prescribed nutrient ratios. Vigilant self-monitoring and intuitive responsiveness to bodily cues are essential. The consultation of healthcare professionals, particularly registered dietitians, is advised for tailored dietary structuring.

10. Perseverance and Sustained Endeavor: The Longitudinal Perspective

The formulation of a balanced dietary regimen for endomorphs transcends transient objectives. The principles of consistency, patience, and gradual progression are pivotal for engendering lasting change, substantiating the transformation into a sustainable lifestyle paradigm.

7 Days Sample Meal Plans for Different Caloric Intakes

here are sample 7-day meal plans for three different caloric intakes: 1500 calories, 2000 calories, and 2500 calories. These meal plans are meant to provide a balanced approach to nutrition and can be adjusted based on individual preferences and dietary needs.

1500-Calorie Meal Plan:

Day 1:

Breakfast: Scrambled eggs with spinach and tomatoes, whole-grain toast

Lunch: Grilled chicken salad with mixed greens, cucumbers, bell peppers, and balsamic vinaigrette

Snack: Greek yogurt with berries

Dinner: Baked salmon, quinoa, and steamed broccoli

Day 2:

Breakfast: Oatmeal topped with sliced banana and almond butter

Lunch: Turkey and avocado wrap with whole-grain tortilla

Snack: Carrot and celery sticks with hummus

Dinner: Stir-fried tofu with mixed vegetables and brown rice

Day 3:

Breakfast: Greek yogurt parfait with granola and mixed berries

Lunch: Chickpea and vegetable soup, whole-grain roll

Snack: Handful of almonds

Dinner: Grilled lean steak, roasted sweet potatoes, and asparagus

Day 4:

Breakfast: Whole-grain pancakes with cottage cheese and sliced strawberries

Lunch: Quinoa and black bean bowl with salsa and avocado

Snack: Apple slices with peanut butter

Dinner: Baked chicken breast, sautéed zucchini, and quinoa

Day 5:

Breakfast: Veggie omelet with whole-grain toast

Lunch: Lentil salad with mixed greens, feta cheese, and vinaigrette

Snack: Cottage cheese with pineapple chunks

Dinner: Grilled fish, steamed green beans, and wild rice

Day 6:

Breakfast: Smoothie with spinach, banana, protein powder, and almond milk

Lunch: Whole-grain pasta salad with vegetables and grilled chicken

Snack: Rice cakes with hummus and cucumber slices

Dinner: Tofu stir-fry with brown rice and snap peas

Day 7:

Breakfast: Whole-grain toast with avocado and poached egg

Lunch: Turkey and vegetable wrap with side salad

Snack: Trail mix with nuts and dried fruits

Dinner: Baked cod, quinoa, and roasted Brussels sprouts

2500-Calorie Meal Plan (Continued):

Day 1:

Breakfast: Veggie-packed omelet with whole-grain toast and avocado

Mid-Morning Snack: Greek yogurt with mixed nuts and honey

Lunch: Grilled chicken breast with quinoa, mixed vegetables, and olive oil dressing

Afternoon Snack: Hummus with whole-grain pita and carrot sticks

Dinner: Salmon fillet, sweet potato mash, and steamed broccoli

Evening Snack: Cottage cheese with fruit and a drizzle of honey

Day 2:

Breakfast: Breakfast burrito with scrambled eggs, black beans, cheese, and salsa

Mid-Morning Snack: Apple slices with almond butter

Lunch: Turkey and avocado salad with mixed greens, nuts, seeds, and balsamic vinaigrette

Afternoon Snack: Trail mix with dried fruits and mixed nuts

Dinner: Grilled steak, quinoa, roasted vegetables, and a side salad

Evening Snack: Greek yogurt with granola and berries

Day 3:

Breakfast: Whole-grain pancakes with a variety of fresh fruits and maple syrup

Mid-Morning Snack: Rice cakes with peanut butter and banana slices

Lunch: Chickpea and vegetable curry with brown rice

Afternoon Snack: Mixed fruit salad with cottage cheese

Dinner: Baked chicken thighs, sweet potato wedges, and asparagus

Evening Snack: Handful of mixed nuts

Day 4:

Breakfast: Smoothie with spinach, banana, berries, protein powder, and almond milk

Mid-Morning Snack: Greek yogurt parfait with granola and mixed nuts

Lunch: Grilled vegetable and hummus wrap with a side salad

Afternoon Snack: Rice cakes with avocado and tomato slices

Dinner: Fish tacos with whole-grain tortillas, coleslaw, and salsa

Evening Snack: Cheese and whole-grain crackers

Day 5:

Breakfast: Scrambled eggs with smoked salmon and whole-grain toast

Mid-Morning Snack: Mixed fruit and cottage cheese

Lunch: Quinoa and black bean salad with avocado, mixed greens, and vinaigrette

Afternoon Snack: Nut butter and banana sandwich on whole-grain bread

Dinner: Grilled shrimp skewers, brown rice, and grilled vegetables

Evening Snack: Handful of trail mix

Day 6:

Breakfast: Oatmeal topped with a variety of nuts, seeds, and dried fruits

Mid-Morning Snack: Greek yogurt with honey and chopped mixed nuts

Lunch: Grilled chicken Caesar salad with whole-grain croutons

Afternoon Snack: Apple slices with cheese

Dinner: Turkey meatballs, whole-grain pasta, marinara sauce, and a side of steamed greens

Evening Snack: Rice cakes with hummus and cucumber slices

Day 7:

Breakfast: Breakfast burrito with scrambled eggs, vegetables, cheese, and salsa

Mid-Morning Snack: Cottage cheese with mixed berries and a drizzle of honey

Lunch: Tuna salad with mixed greens, olives, cherry tomatoes, and olive oil dressing

Afternoon Snack: Whole-grain crackers with guacamole

Dinner: Stir-fried tofu with vegetables, brown rice, and teriyaki sauce

Evening Snack: Greek yogurt with chopped nuts and a sprinkle of cinnamon

2000-Calorie Meal Plan:

Day 1:

Breakfast: Scrambled eggs with sautéed spinach and whole-grain toast

Lunch: Grilled chicken salad with mixed greens, cherry tomatoes, cucumbers, and vinaigrette

Snack: Greek yogurt with a handful of mixed berries

Dinner: Baked salmon with quinoa and roasted asparagus

Day 2:

Breakfast: Whole-grain oatmeal topped with sliced bananas, chopped nuts, and a drizzle of honey

Lunch: Turkey and avocado wrap with whole-grain tortilla and a side salad

Snack: Carrot and celery sticks with hummus

Dinner: Stir-fried tofu with broccoli, bell peppers, and brown rice

Day 3:

Breakfast: Greek yogurt parfait with granola and assorted fruits

Lunch: Lentil and vegetable soup with a whole-grain roll

Snack: Handful of almonds

Dinner: Grilled chicken breast with sweet potato mash and steamed green beans

Day 4:

Breakfast: Smoothie with mixed berries, spinach, protein powder, and almond milk

Lunch: Chickpea and quinoa salad with mixed vegetables and a lemon-tahini dressing

Snack: Apple slices with almond butter

Dinner: Baked fish with roasted vegetables and wild rice

Day 5:

Breakfast: Whole-grain toast with avocado and a poached egg

Lunch: Turkey and vegetable stir-fry with brown rice

Snack: Cottage cheese with pineapple chunks

Dinner: Grilled lean steak with a side of quinoa and steamed broccoli

Day 6:

Breakfast: Veggie omelet with feta cheese and whole-grain toast

Lunch: Hummus and grilled vegetable wrap with a side of mixed greens

Snack: Mixed nuts and dried fruits

Dinner: Baked chicken thighs with quinoa and sautéed spinach

Day 7:

Breakfast: Whole-grain pancakes with mixed berries and a dollop of Greek yogurt

Lunch: Quinoa and black bean bowl with avocado, salsa, and a side salad

Snack: Rice cakes with peanut butter

Dinner: Grilled fish with a side of roasted sweet potatoes and Brussels sprouts

Meal Timing and Frequency for Optimal Results

Meal frequency and timing are important factors in maximizing your nutrition and reaching your health and fitness objectives. Tailoring your eating routine to your requirements and objectives can aid in energy regulation, metabolic support, and general well-being. Here's a breakdown of ideal meal timing and frequency:

Understanding the Significance of Meal Timing and Frequency

The timing and frequency of our meals constitute crucial aspects of our dietary habits that profoundly impact our metabolic and physiological processes. The strategic alignment of meals throughout the day holds the potential to influence energy levels, metabolic efficiency, and overall well-being. Delving into the intricacies of meal timing and frequency can provide valuable insights into how to harness these factors to our advantage.

1. Breakfast: Igniting the Metabolic Furnace

Commencing the day with a well-balanced breakfast emerges as an essential practice. Breakfast serves as the metaphorical spark that kindles our metabolic furnace, catalyzing energy production and initiating the cascade of biochemical reactions that underpin physiological activities. A breakfast rich in protein, complex carbohydrates, and healthy fats cultivates a foundation of sustained energy release.

2. Mid-Morning Snack: Maintaining Energy Equilibrium

A mid-morning snack presents itself as a strategic maneuver, particularly if the interval between breakfast and lunch is considerable. This interlude functions to sustain energy equilibrium and mitigate potential energy lulls. Opting for a snack comprising protein and fiber fosters satiety and serves as a nutritional bridge until the subsequent meal.

3. Lunch: Nutrient Replenishment and Sustenance

Lunch assumes the role of a pivotal interlude, providing the opportunity to replenish nutrients and sustain physiological homeostasis. A judiciously balanced lunch characterizes itself by the amalgamation of lean proteins, complex carbohydrates, and wholesome fats. This composition engenders a surge of sustained energy, fortifying cognitive function and physical stamina.

4. Afternoon Snack: Tempering Afternoon Fatigue

As the afternoon progresses, the inclusion of an afternoon snack can circumvent the onset of fatigue and prevent excessive hunger, which may culminate in overindulgence during dinner. Opting for a snack that unites protein and fiber cultivates satiety, while also steering clear of rapid blood sugar fluctuations.

5. Dinner: Culmination of Nourishment

Dinner represents the culmination of daily nourishment, necessitating a judicious orchestration of nutrients to satiate both physiological requirements and sensory gratification. Akin to lunch, dinner ought to encompass lean proteins, complex carbohydrates, and abundant vegetables. Allowing for a modest temporal gap between dinner and sleep facilitates optimal digestion and sleep quality.

6. Evening Snack (Optional): Mindful Choices

Should the occasion arise, an evening snack can be a prudent option, provided it aligns with the principles of portion control and nutrient density. Selections like cottage cheese paired with fruit or a modest portion of whole-grain cereal exhibit characteristics of satiety and nutritional prudence.

Tailoring Meal Frequency: A Customized Approach

The frequency of meals and snacks warrants individualized calibration. Preferences, activity levels, and personal circadian rhythms guide this customization. This can range from a three-meal paradigm to an extended structure encompassing five to six smaller meals and snacks. The objective is to achieve a pattern that optimally sustains energy levels and aligns with one's lifestyle.

Holistic Hydration: A Fundamental Underpinning

Beyond sustenance, the theme of hydration assumes centrality. Consistent water intake throughout the day is pivotal for metabolic vigor, nutrient transportation, and physiological equilibrium. Adequate hydration complements the rhythm of nourishment.

Mindful Eating: A Contemplative Approach

Amid the orchestration of meal timing and frequency, the practice of mindful eating emerges as an indispensable companion. Consciously attending to hunger cues, savoring each morsel, and cultivating an attuned relationship with our body's signals engenders a wholesome eating experience.

CHAPTER 5

IMPLEMENTING METABOLIC CONFUSION WORKOUTS

The Marriage of Diet and Exercise: Why Both Matter

Imagine diet and exercise as two dance partners on a health journey, moving in sync to create a mesmerizing choreography of well-being. These seemingly distinct elements share an intimate connection that goes beyond mere coexistence. Let's dive into why this dynamic duo matters so much, unveiling their intertwined significance.

1. Dynamic Duo for Weight Management

Think of diet and exercise as the ultimate tag team for weight management. A well-balanced diet helps regulate calorie intake, while exercise burns those calories, creating a harmonious calorie balance. This collaboration becomes a potent strategy for weight loss or maintaining a healthy weight.

2. Sculpting Muscles Through Collaboration

Diet and exercise engage in a fascinating tango when it comes to muscles. Your diet's protein content serves as the building blocks for muscle repair and growth. Exercise, especially strength training, then steps in to trigger muscle fibers to adapt and flourish.

3. Metabolism: A Symphony of Efficiency

The synergy of diet and exercise orchestrates a metabolic symphony. A nourishing diet fuels metabolic processes, ensuring nutrients are readily available for energy production. Simultaneously, regular exercise elevates metabolic rate, optimizing energy utilization and tapping into fat stores for fuel.

4. Hormones and Harmony

Picture diet and exercise as the maestros of hormone balance. A diet rich in nutrients like healthy fats and complex carbs supports hormone production. Meanwhile, exercise unleashes endorphins and other mood-elevating hormones, enhancing emotional equilibrium.

5. Heart Health: A Pas de Deux

Diet and exercise perform a mesmerizing duet for cardiovascular health. A heart-loving diet, packed with fiber, antioxidants, and omega-3s, supports blood pressure and cholesterol levels. At the same time, exercise polishes the heart's performance, enhancing circulation and guarding against heart diseases.

6. Mental Agility: A Choreography of Clarity

The interplay of diet and exercise extends its influence on mental agility. Nutrient-dense diets provide the brain's building blocks, while physical activity pumps up cerebral blood flow, enhancing cognitive prowess.

7. Lifelong Vibrancy

The fusion of diet and exercise becomes an elixir for longevity and disease prevention. A nourishing diet, coupled with regular exercise, acts as a shield against chronic illnesses, empowering individuals to embrace vibrant health throughout their lives.

8. Serenade to Well-Being

This synergistic dance touches the strings of psychological well-being. Wholesome diets foster neurotransmitter production, influencing mood. Physical activity, especially mindful practices, emerges as a stress-busting rhythm, nurturing mental resilience.

9. Custom Choreography for Goals

Recognizing the partnership of diet and exercise means personalizing your routine to your aspirations. You can tailor your dietary choices and exercise routines to align with specific goals, whether it's shedding pounds, gaining muscle, or just embracing overall vitality.

Customizing Workouts for Endomorph Women

Designing exercise routines tailored to the unique characteristics of endomorph women necessitates a comprehensive understanding of their physiological traits. Endomorphs tend to possess a higher proportion of body fat and a relatively slower metabolic rate. Nonetheless, this distinctive makeup doesn't preclude achieving fitness objectives; rather, it underscores the significance of crafting personalized workout plans that resonate harmoniously with their body composition. Let's delve into the intricate process of formulating exercise regimens that cater to the specific needs of endomorph women:

1. Cardiovascular Exercise with Intervals: Cardiovascular exercises emerge as an essential component for caloric expenditure and cardiovascular health. For endomorph women, interval training emerges as a strategic choice. This approach integrates brief periods of high-intensity exercises, such as sprints or plyometric movements, followed by brief intervals of low-intensity recovery. By embracing this approach, endomorphs can optimize calorie burn, stimulate metabolism, and circumvent adaptation.

2. Emphasis on Strength Training:

Strength training stands as a cornerstone for bolstering metabolic rate and refining physique contours. Prioritize compound movements like squats, deadlifts, and lunges, which activate multiple muscle groups concurrently. Striving for moderate to substantial resistance levels while progressively intensifying the load empowers endomorph women to foster muscle growth and metabolic efficiency.

3. Harnessing Resistance Training:

Leveraging resistance bands or bodyweight exercises can facilitate the cultivation of lean muscle mass. This becomes instrumental in augmenting metabolic activity and facilitating fat loss—a crucial consideration for endomorphs seeking optimal body composition.

4. Leveraging High-Intensity Interval Training (HIIT):

HIIT workouts present an enticing avenue for endomorph women due to their remarkable potential for elevating metabolism and fat oxidation. By intertwining brief bursts of vigorous activity with short recovery intervals, HIIT stimulates the body's physiological responses, propelling calorie expenditure and post-exercise benefits.

5. Embrace Circuit Training:

Circuit training, an amalgamation of cardiovascular and strength-based exercises sequenced in rapid succession, offers a comprehensive workout strategy. This approach engenders an elevated calorie burn, enhances muscular endurance, and fosters cardiovascular fitness, making it an apt choice for endomorphs aspiring for fat loss and muscle refinement.

6. Cultivating Flexibility and Mobility:

Prioritizing flexibility and mobility interventions, encompassing practices like yoga or Pilates contributes to holistic well-being. These modalities enhance joint flexibility, alleviate stress, and expedite post-workout recovery, making them a valuable inclusion in the regimen.

7. Revering Rest and Recovery:

Endomorph women should allocate due importance to restorative days to forestall overtraining and promote muscular recuperation. Prioritizing adequate sleep, sound nutritional choices and active recovery techniques such as foam rolling fosters a balanced workout routine.

8. Personalized Nutrition:

Considering that endomorphs may be predisposed to weight gain, a meticulous dietary approach is imperative. Prioritize a nutrient-rich diet featuring whole foods, lean protein sources, healthy fats, and complex carbohydrates. Portion control is pivotal, and meals should be attuned to energy expenditure and fitness objectives.

9. The Role of Consistency:

Sustained consistency stands as the linchpin of accomplishing fitness goals. Endomorph women must commit to regular exercise sessions and a well-balanced nutritional regime over time to unveil sustainable transformations.

10. Engage Professional Expertise:

Collaborating with a certified fitness professional or a registered dietitian, well-versed in the nuances of endomorph body types, is a prudent step. These experts can guide the creation of a bespoke exercise and dietary blueprint that harmonizes with individual aspirations, constraints, and preferences.

CHAPTER 6

OVERCOMING CHALLENGES AND STAYING CONSISTENT

Dealing with Cravings and Emotional Eating

The intricate landscape of cravings and emotional eating is a common terrain to tread, yet with the right insights and strategies, it's entirely manageable. These tendencies can sometimes lead us astray from our nutritional goals, but by delving into the dynamics at play and applying effective approaches, you can regain control over your eating habits. Here's a comprehensive guide to gracefully navigate cravings and emotional eating:

1. Decode Trigger Points: Start by deciphering the triggers that set off your cravings and emotional eating episodes. These triggers could be stress, monotony, sadness, or the environments you find yourself in. Illuminating these triggers allows you to preemptively manage them.

2. Discern Hunger from Cravings: Distinguish the nuances between genuine physical hunger and emotional cravings. When the urge to eat arises, pause and reflect on whether your body truly needs sustenance or if it's an emotional impulse. This awareness is a powerful tool in curbing emotional eating.

3. Embrace Mindful Eating: Infuse mindfulness into your eating routine. This involves immersing yourself fully in the sensory experience of your meals. Engage your senses, relish each bite, and savor the textures and flavors. This practice heightens your connection to your body's cues of hunger and fullness.

4. Holistic Emotional Coping: Instead of utilizing food as an emotional refuge, explore diverse avenues for managing emotions. Engage in activities that resonate with you, whether it's exercising, meditating, painting, or simply unwinding with a book. These alternatives provide constructive outlets for emotional release.

5. Blueprint Balanced Meals: Craft a culinary blueprint that champions balance. Ensure your meals comprise a medley of nutrients – protein, healthy fats, and complex carbohydrates. This nutritional equilibrium stabilizes blood sugar levels, curbing intense cravings.

6. Out of Sight, Out of Mind: Minimize the temptation by keeping trigger foods out of sight. Opt for healthier alternatives that are readily accessible, thereby nudging your choices in a positive direction.

7. Hydration, the Silent Ally: Dehydration often disguises itself as hunger or cravings. Uphold your hydration levels with ample water intake throughout the day, diminishing the likelihood of needless snacking.

8. Portion Mastery: Should you choose to indulge in a craving, do so mindfully and with moderation. Portion control is a wise ally in the quest to manage cravings without derailing your goals.

9. Anticipatory Snacking: When venturing into situations that might trigger cravings, preemptively partake in a wholesome snack. This pre-emptive measure safeguards against ravenous hunger and impulsive choices.

10. Forge a Support System: Open up about your journey to a confidant – be it a friend, family member, or counselor. A support system offers encouragement, accountability, and a cushion during challenging moments.

11. Chronicle in a Food Diary: Document your eating patterns, emotions, and triggers in a journal. This reflective exercise unveils patterns and empowers you to make informed decisions to address emotional eating.

12. Cultivate Self-Compassion: Embrace self-kindness and acknowledge that slips are part of the journey. Instead of fixating on mistakes, focus on the progressive choices you can make going forward.

13. Professional Guidance: If emotional eating persists as a formidable challenge, consider seeking guidance from a registered dietitian or therapist. Their expertise equips you with tailored strategies to address the underlying emotional currents.

Navigating Social Situations and Dining Out

Embarking on a journey towards healthier eating need not entail retreating from social engagements or dining experiences. With a methodical approach and prudent planning, you can relish social occasions while harmonizing with your wellness aspirations. Here's an instructive guide on skillfully navigating social situations and dining out:

1. Preemptive Menu Evaluation:

Before venturing out to dine, take a proactive step by perusing the menu online, if available. This proactive measure empowers you to make informed choices in advance, mitigating impulsive decisions at the table.

2. Prudent Venue Selection:

Opt for dining establishments that offer a diverse array of nourishing options on their menu. This expands your scope of choices and encourages health-conscious selections without feeling constrained.

3. Conscientious Ordering:

When placing your order, favor preparations like grilling, baking, or steaming over fried or heavily sautéed alternatives. Request dressings and sauces to be served on the side, granting you authority over portion control.

4. Portion Awareness:

It's worth noting that restaurant portion sizes often exceed typical requirements. Contemplate sharing an entrée with a companion, selecting a smaller portion, or setting aside half your meal for a later occasion.

5. Embrace Vegetable Abundance:

Prioritize dishes enriched with vegetables, whole grains, and lean protein sources. These nutrient-rich selections satiate hunger and supply essential nutrients.

6. Beverage Management:

Elevate your beverage acumen by favoring water, unsweetened tea, or sparkling water. Limit consumption of sugary beverages and alcohol, which can introduce surplus calories devoid of substantial nutritional value.

7. Prelude of Social Interaction:

Prioritize engaging in conversation and social interaction before initiating your meal. This deliberate approach allows your body to register authentic hunger cues, preempting overindulgence stemming from distractions.

8. Mindful Gastronomy:

Embark on the practice of mindful eating, characterized by savoring each morsel, chewing with deliberation, and intermittently placing utensils aside. This fosters a heightened connection with your nourishment, thwarting hastiness.

9. Indulgence with Intention:

Should a treat or dessert beckon, indulge with purpose and awareness. Immerse yourself in the experience, relishing each bite, and attuning to your body's responses.

10. Stratagem for Special Occasions:

For momentous events, strategize by moderating your intake throughout the day. Opt for lighter fare before and following the event, creating room for indulgence while upholding equilibrium.

11. Communicate Assertively:

Don't shy away from articulating your dietary preferences or requirements to companions or the server. Many dining establishments are amenable to customization.

12. Cultivate Mindful Social Pursuits:

Cultivate social endeavors that transcend the realm of food. Suggest activities such as walks, museum visits, or other engaging experiences that foster interaction sans a culinary focus.

13. Shift of Center:

Steer the spotlight away from food and onto the enriching camaraderie and discourse. Engaging in conversations and authentic connections can relegate the meal to a secondary role.

14. Embrace Adaptive Mindset:

Remember that occasional indulgence is not only permissible but also conducive to balance. Approach these moments with a focus on progress rather than an unrealistic pursuit of flawlessness.

15. Uplifting Perspective:

Infuse your dining-out experiences with a positive lens. View them as opportunities to exercise mindfulness and aligned choices that resonate with your holistic well-being.

Tracking Progress: Beyond the Scale

When embarking on a journey to improve health and fitness, it's important to recognize that progress cannot be solely measured by the numbers on a scale. While weight is an observable marker, a comprehensive assessment takes into account various dimensions. Here's an overview of tracking progress beyond the scale, encompassing both physical and non-physical aspects:

1. Body Measurements: Regularly measuring key body areas, such as the waist, hips, chest, and limbs, provides insight into changes in body composition. Reductions in measurements can signify changes in fat and muscle proportions, even if weight remains stable.

2. Body Composition Analysis: Methods like bioelectrical impedance or DEXA scans offer a breakdown of body fat and lean muscle mass. This data provides a more accurate depiction of your body's composition changes.

3. Fitness Levels: Monitoring improvements in fitness capabilities is crucial. Progress may manifest in running longer distances, lifting heavier weights, or achieving more advanced yoga poses, reflecting enhanced strength, endurance, and flexibility.

4. Energy Levels: Heightened energy levels and reduced fatigue in daily activities are indicators of improved fitness and overall well-being.

5. Mood and Mental Well-being: Positive shifts in mood, decreased stress levels, and improved mental clarity are significant markers of progress. Regular exercise is known to have a positive impact on mental health.

6. Sleep Quality: Observing improvements in sleep patterns, such as falling asleep more easily, experiencing fewer interruptions, and waking up feeling rejuvenated, signifies positive changes.

7. Clothing Fit: Changes in how your clothes fit or the need to opt for smaller sizes reflect shifts in body composition, even if the scale doesn't show drastic changes.

8. Performance Enhancements: If you engage in athletic pursuits, track enhancements in performance, such as achieving faster race times, increased endurance, or refined athletic skills.

9. Health Risk Factors: Consistent exercise and a balanced diet contribute to better health markers, including improved blood pressure, cholesterol levels, and blood sugar control.

10. Digestive Health: Positive changes in digestion, reduced bloating, and an overall improvement in gut health can be attributed to dietary adjustments and increased physical activity.

11. Self-Confidence: As you witness progress and positive changes, your self-esteem and body confidence often experience a boost.

12. Consistency and Habits: Monitoring your ability to maintain a regular exercise routine and adhere to healthy habits is a significant accomplishment. Consistency is a fundamental factor in achieving sustainable results.

13. Lifestyle Changes: Shifts towards healthier lifestyle habits, such as cooking more at home, opting for nutrient-rich foods, and practicing mindful eating, indicate a positive transformation.

14. Functional Fitness: The ability to carry out everyday tasks with greater ease – lifting groceries, ascending stairs, or engaging in physical activities – signifies enhanced functional fitness.

15. Social Support and Accountability: Building a network of support and accountability, whether through friends, family, or fitness communities, contributes to an environment conducive to progress.

CHAPTER 7

MEAL PREPPING AND RECIPES FOR SUCCESS

The Role of Meal Prepping in Sustained Success

Meal prepping stands as a strategic and proactive approach to meal management that holds significant importance in securing sustained success on your journey toward health and fitness. By dedicating time to plan, prepare, and organize your meals ahead of time, you unlock a range of benefits that contribute profoundly to your enduring well-being and fitness aspirations. Here's an educational breakdown of the role of meal prepping in fostering long-term success:

1. Consistency in Nutritional Intake: Meal prepping empowers you to align with balanced nutrition consistently. The act of planning your meals meticulously helps you make thoughtful dietary choices, curbing the tendency to opt for less nourishing options impulsively.

2. Mastering Portion Control: At the heart of wholesome eating lies portion control. Meal prepping facilitates this practice by enabling you to measure and portion your meals accurately, thereby preventing excessive consumption. This mindful approach fosters an understanding of appropriate portion sizes and aids in regulating calorie intake.

3. Efficiency and Convenience in Time Management: In the fast-paced contemporary world, carving out time for daily cooking can be challenging. Meal prepping counters this hurdle by front-loading the culinary effort. It grants you the luxury of time during busy days, as your meals are prepared in advance and at your disposal.

4. Taming Impulse Choices: Moments of hunger and time constraints often lead to hasty, unhealthy food choices. By prepping your meals, you secure a repertoire of healthier alternatives that are readily available, thus diminishing the temptation to veer toward less nutritious options.

5. Financial Prudence: Frequent dining out can strain your budget. Engaging in meal prepping allows you to harness the economics of bulk buying, resulting in long-term savings. Furthermore, the cost of prepared meals often proves more economical than restaurant expenditures.

6. Empowerment Over Ingredients: Meal prepping places you at the helm of ingredient selection. This autonomy enables you to opt for fresh, high-quality components, regulate seasoning and serving sizes, and circumvent excess sugars, unhealthy fats, and additives.

7. Upholding Dietary Consistency: Irrespective of whether you adhere to a specific dietary regimen or pursue certain macronutrient ratios, meal prepping becomes an invaluable ally in maintaining steadfast consistency. When your meals align with your dietary objectives, the likelihood of adherence increases.

8. Liberation from Decision Fatigue: The daily array of food-related choices can exert cognitive strain. Meal prepping alleviates the burden of spontaneous decision-making, liberating mental bandwidth for other cognitive demands.

9. Catering to Special Dietary Needs: For those with dietary restrictions, allergies, or distinct health targets, meal prepping furnishes a platform for customization. You can accommodate specific needs without sacrificing flavor or variety.

10. Support for Active Schedules: Individuals entrenched in demanding routines find solace in meal prepping. It ensures that nutritionally balanced meals remain accessible, even during hectic stretches where conventional cooking might be unfeasible.

11. Cultivation of Mindful Eating: With pre-prepared meals, you're poised to engage in mindful consumption. This practice encourages savoring each bite, fostering a deeper connection with your nourishment and promoting optimal digestion.

12. Curbing Food Waste: Meal prepping contributes to resourcefulness and curbs food wastage. Ingredients are employed efficiently, and leftovers can be repurposed for subsequent meals.

Quick and Nutrient-Dense Recipe Ideas

Greek Yogurt Parfait:

Ingredients:

1 cup Greek yogurt (low-fat or non-fat)

1/2 cup mixed berries (blueberries, strawberries, raspberries)

1 tablespoon honey or maple syrup

2 tablespoons granola

Instructions:

In a glass or bowl, layer Greek yogurt, mixed berries, and granola.

Drizzle honey or maple syrup over the top.

Enjoy your creamy and protein-packed parfait!

Nutritional Information (approximate):

Calories: 250

Protein: 15g

Carbohydrates: 40g

Fiber: 4g

Fat: 4g

Avocado Toast with Egg:

Ingredients:

1 slice whole-grain bread, toasted

1/2 avocado, mashed

1 egg, cooked (fried, scrambled, or poached)

Salt and pepper to taste

Optional toppings: red pepper flakes, chopped herbs

Instructions:

Spread mashed avocado on the toasted bread.

Top with cooked egg.

Sprinkle with salt, pepper, and any optional toppings you prefer.

Nutritional Information (approximate):

Calories: 300

Protein: 13g

Carbohydrates: 22g

Fiber: 8g

Fat: 18g

Oatmeal with Nut Butter and Banana:

Ingredients:

1/2 cup rolled oats

1 cup milk (dairy or plant-based)

1 tablespoon nut butter (peanut, almond, etc.)

1/2 banana, sliced

1 teaspoon chia seeds (optional)

Cinnamon for flavor

Instructions:

Cook oats in milk according to package instructions.

Top with nut butter, banana slices, chia seeds, and a sprinkle of cinnamon.

Nutritional Information (approximate):

Calories: 380

Protein: 12g

Carbohydrates: 50g

Fiber: 8g

Fat: 15g

Veggie and Cheese Omelette:

Ingredients:

2 eggs

1/4 cup diced bell peppers

1/4 cup diced tomatoes

1/4 cup chopped spinach

1/4 cup shredded cheese (cheddar, mozzarella, etc.)

Salt, pepper, and herbs for seasoning

Instructions:

In a bowl, whisk eggs and season with salt and pepper.

In a non-stick pan, sauté bell peppers, tomatoes, and spinach until slightly softened.

Pour whisked eggs over the veggies, and cook until set.

Sprinkle shredded cheese on one half, fold the omelet, and cook until the cheese melts.

Nutritional Information (approximate):

Calories: 280

Protein: 20g

Carbohydrates: 7g

Fiber: 2g

Fat: 19g

Smoothie Bowl:

Ingredients:

1 frozen banana

1/2 cup frozen mixed berries

1/2 cup spinach or kale

1/2 cup milk (dairy or plant-based)

1 tablespoon nut butter

Toppings: granola, sliced fruits, nuts, seeds

Instructions:

Blend frozen banana, mixed berries, spinach or kale, milk, and nut butter until smooth.

Pour the smoothie into a bowl.

Top with granola, sliced fruits, nuts, and seeds.

Nutritional Information (approximate):

Calories: 350

Protein: 10g

Carbohydrates: 55g

Fiber: 9g

Fat: 13g

Quinoa Salad with Chickpeas and Veggies:

Ingredients:

1 cup cooked quinoa

1 cup canned chickpeas, drained and rinsed

1 cup diced cucumber

1 cup diced bell peppers

1/4 cup chopped fresh parsley

2 tablespoons feta cheese (optional)

2 tablespoons olive oil

Juice of 1 lemon

Salt and pepper to taste

Instructions: In a large bowl, combine cooked quinoa, chickpeas, cucumber, bell peppers, and parsley.

In a small bowl, whisk together olive oil, lemon juice, salt, and pepper.

Pour the dressing over the quinoa mixture and toss well.

Sprinkle feta cheese on top if desired.

Nutritional Information (approximate):

Calories: 400

Protein: 12g

Carbohydrates: 55g

Fiber: 10g

Fat: 16g

Grilled Chicken Wrap with Hummus and Veggies:

Ingredients:

1 whole wheat wrap or tortilla

4 oz grilled chicken breast, sliced

2 tablespoons hummus

1/2 cup sliced tomatoes

1/2 cup sliced cucumbers

1/4 cup shredded lettuce

Salt and pepper to taste

Instructions:

Lay the wrap flat and spread the hummus evenly.

Place sliced grilled chicken, tomatoes, cucumbers, and shredded lettuce on top.

Season with salt and pepper.

Roll up the wrap tightly and enjoy.

Nutritional Information (approximate):

Calories: 350

Protein: 30g

Carbohydrates: 35g

Fiber: 7g

Fat: 10g

Lentil and Vegetable Stir-Fry:

Ingredients:

1 cup cooked green or brown lentils

1 cup mixed stir-fry vegetables (broccoli, carrots, bell peppers)

1 tablespoon olive oil

2 tablespoons low-sodium soy sauce

1 clove garlic, minced

1 teaspoon grated ginger

Crushed red pepper flakes (optional)

Sesame seeds for garnish

Instructions: In a pan, heat olive oil over medium heat.

Add minced garlic and grated ginger, and sauté for a minute.

Add stir-fry vegetables and cook until slightly tender.

Stir in cooked lentils and soy sauce. Add red pepper flakes if desired.

Cook for another few minutes until heated through.

Garnish with sesame seeds before serving.

Nutritional Information (approximate):

Calories: 350

Protein: 20g

Carbohydrates: 50g

Fiber: 15g

Fat: 8g

Spinach and Chickpea Salad with Tuna:

Ingredients:

2 cups baby spinach

1/2 cup canned chickpeas, drained and rinsed

1 can tuna, drained

1/4 cup diced red onion

1/4 cup diced cucumber

2 tablespoons balsamic vinaigrette

Salt and pepper to taste

Instructions: In a large bowl, combine baby spinach, chickpeas, tuna, red onion, and cucumber.

Drizzle balsamic vinaigrette over the salad.

Season with salt and pepper.

Toss well and enjoy your refreshing salad.

Nutritional Information (approximate):

Calories: 300

Protein: 30g

Carbohydrates: 20g

Fiber: 5g

Fat: 10g

Vegetable and Quinoa Stir-Fry:

Ingredients:

1 cup cooked quinoa

1 cup mixed stir-fry vegetables (zucchini, carrots, snap peas)

1 tablespoon sesame oil

2 tablespoons low-sodium soy sauce

1 tablespoon rice vinegar

1 teaspoon honey

1/2 teaspoon grated ginger

Sesame seeds for garnish

Instructions:

In a pan, heat sesame oil over medium heat.

Add stir-fry vegetables and sauté until crisp-tender.

In a small bowl, whisk together soy sauce, rice vinegar, honey, and grated ginger.

Add cooked quinoa to the pan and pour the sauce over the vegetables and quinoa.

Stir-fry for a couple of minutes until well combined.

Garnish with sesame seeds before serving.

Nutritional Information (approximate):

Calories: 350

Protein: 10g

Carbohydrates: 50g

Fiber: 8g

Fat: 12g

Baked Salmon with Roasted Vegetables:

Ingredients:

1 salmon fillet (6 oz)

1 cup mixed vegetables (broccoli, carrots, bell peppers)

1 tablespoon olive oil

Lemon zest and juice

Salt, pepper, and herbs for seasoning

Instructions: Preheat the oven to 400°F (200°C).

Place salmon on a baking sheet and drizzle with olive oil, lemon zest, and juice.

Season with salt, pepper, and herbs.

Arrange mixed vegetables around the salmon.

Bake for about 15-20 minutes or until the salmon is cooked and flakes easily with a fork.

Nutritional Information (approximate):

Calories: 400

Protein: 30g

Carbohydrates: 15g

Fiber: 5g

Fat: 25g

Chickpea and Vegetable Stir-Fry with Brown Rice:

Ingredients:

1 cup cooked brown rice

1 cup canned chickpeas, drained and rinsed

1 cup mixed stir-fry vegetables (snow peas, carrots, bell peppers)

2 tablespoons low-sodium soy sauce

1 tablespoon sesame oil

1 teaspoon minced garlic

Crushed red pepper flakes (optional)

Instructions: Heat sesame oil in a pan over medium heat.

Add minced garlic and stir-fry vegetables. Cook until tender.

Add chickpeas and cooked brown rice to the pan.

Pour soy sauce over the mixture and add red pepper flakes if desired.

Stir-fry for a few minutes until well combined and heated through.

Nutritional Information (approximate):

Calories: 450

Protein: 14g

Carbohydrates: 70g

Fiber: 12g

Fat: 14g

Grilled Chicken with Quinoa and Steamed Broccoli:

Ingredients:

4 oz grilled chicken breast

1/2 cup cooked quinoa

1 cup steamed broccoli

1 tablespoon olive oil

Lemon juice

Salt, pepper, and herbs for seasoning

Instructions: Season grilled chicken with olive oil, lemon juice, salt, pepper, and herbs.

Serve the grilled chicken with cooked quinoa and steamed broccoli on the side.

Nutritional Information (approximate):

Calories: 400

Protein: 30g

Carbohydrates: 30g

Fiber: 5g

Fat: 15g

Lentil and Spinach Salad with Feta:

Ingredients:

1 cup cooked green lentils

2 cups baby spinach

1/4 cup crumbled feta cheese

1/4 cup diced red onion

1/4 cup diced cucumber

2 tablespoons balsamic vinaigrette

Salt and pepper to taste

Instructions: In a large bowl, combine cooked lentils, baby spinach, feta cheese, red onion, and cucumber.

Drizzle balsamic vinaigrette over the salad.

Season with salt and pepper.

Toss well and enjoy your nutritious salad.

Nutritional Information (approximate):

Calories: 350

Protein: 18g

Carbohydrates: 40g

Fiber: 15g

Fat: 12g

Veggie and Tofu Stir-Fry with Noodles:

Ingredients: 1 cup cooked whole wheat or rice noodles

4 oz firm tofu, cubed

1 cup mixed stir-fry vegetables (bok choy, carrots, bell peppers)

2 tablespoons low-sodium soy sauce

1 tablespoon hoisin sauce

1 teaspoon sesame oil

1 teaspoon minced ginger

Chopped green onions for garnish

Instructions: In a pan, heat sesame oil over medium heat.

Add cubed tofu and stir-fry until lightly browned.

Add minced ginger and mixed vegetables. Cook until vegetables are tender.

Stir in cooked noodles, soy sauce, and hoisin sauce.

Cook for a few minutes until heated through.

Garnish with chopped green onions before serving.

Nutritional Information (approximate):

Calories: 400

Protein: 15g

Carbohydrates: 55g

Fiber: 8g

Fat: 12g

Greek Yogurt Parfait with Berries and Nuts:

Ingredients:

1/2 cup Greek yogurt (low-fat or non-fat)

1/4 cup mixed berries (blueberries, strawberries, raspberries)

1 tablespoon chopped nuts (almonds, walnuts)

1 teaspoon honey or maple syrup

Instructions:

In a glass or bowl, layer Greek yogurt, mixed berries, and chopped nuts.

Drizzle honey or maple syrup over the top.

Enjoy your creamy and protein-rich parfait!

Nutritional Information (approximate):

Calories: 200

Protein: 12g

Carbohydrates: 20g

Fiber: 3g

Fat: 8g

Dark Chocolate-Dipped Strawberries:

Ingredients:

6 fresh strawberries

2 oz dark chocolate (70% cocoa or higher)

Instructions: Melt dark chocolate in a microwave-safe bowl in 20-second intervals, stirring in between.

Dip each strawberry into the melted chocolate, covering half of the strawberry.

Place the dipped strawberries on a parchment-lined tray and let the chocolate set in the refrigerator.

Enjoy your delicious and antioxidant-rich treat!

Nutritional Information (approximate):

Calories: 150

Protein: 2g

Carbohydrates: 18g

Fiber: 4g

Fat: 9g

Frozen Banana Bites:

Ingredients:

1 ripe banana, sliced

2 tablespoons nut butter (peanut, almond)

2 tablespoons dark chocolate chips

Instructions: Spread nut butter on one side of banana slices.

Sandwich two banana slices together with nut butter in the middle.

Dip each banana sandwich into melted dark chocolate.

Place on a tray lined with parchment paper and freeze until the chocolate sets.

Enjoy your frozen, creamy delight!

Nutritional Information (approximate):

Calories: 200

Protein: 4g

Carbohydrates: 30g

Fiber: 4g

Fat: 9g

Chia Seed Pudding with Mixed Berries:

Ingredients:

2 tablespoons chia seeds

1/2 cup unsweetened almond milk (or any milk of choice)

1/2 teaspoon vanilla extract

1/4 cup mixed berries (blueberries, raspberries)

Instructions: In a bowl, mix chia seeds, almond milk, and vanilla extract.

Stir well and let it sit in the refrigerator for at least 2 hours or overnight to thicken.

Top with mixed berries before serving.

Enjoy your fiber-rich and omega-3-packed dessert!

Nutritional Information (approximate):

Calories: 150

Protein: 4g

Carbohydrates: 16g

Fiber: 10g

Fat: 8g

Baked Apple with Cinnamon and Greek Yogurt:

Ingredients:

1 medium apple

1 teaspoon cinnamon

2 tablespoons Greek yogurt (low-fat or non-fat)

Instructions:

Preheat the oven to 350°F (175°C).

Core the apple and place it in a baking dish.

Sprinkle cinnamon over the apple.

Bake for about 20-25 minutes or until the apple is soft.

Top with Greek yogurt before serving.

Enjoy your warm and comforting dessert!

Nutritional Information (approximate):

Calories: 150

Protein: 4g

Carbohydrates: 35g

Fiber: 6g

Fat: 1g

Cooking Tips and Grocery Shopping for Your Metabolic Confusion Diet

Efficiently navigating the tenets of the Metabolic Confusion Diet necessitates a profound understanding not only of its foundational principles but also the astute management of grocery procurement and culinary endeavors. In light of this, here we elucidate a compendium of cooking strategies and discerning guidelines for effective grocery acquisitions that harmonize seamlessly with the precepts of the Metabolic Confusion Diet:

Culinary Strategies:

- Preparatory Alacrity: It is judicious to allocate a portion of each week for meticulous meal planning and culinary preemption. Slicing and dicing vegetables, marinating proteins, and precooking essentials like quinoa or brown rice can streamline moments of culinary exigency, thereby imbuing temporal efficacy.

- Communal Repast Production: Cultivating the practice of culinary mass production is pragmatic. Preparing sizable quantities of specific repasts that exhibit malleability across various days is a potent stratagem. For instance, envisage orchestrating an ample assemblage of grilled chicken or roasted vegetables that bestows versatility to diverse culinary manifestations throughout the temporal sphere.

- Optimal Protein Selection: Prudently select lean protein sources, such as turkey, skinless poultry, lean beef cuts, fish, tofu, and tempeh. These substrates are sine qua non for the preservation of lean muscle mass and facilitation of metabolism.

- Vivid Vegetable Spectrum: Embrace a mélange of vibrant vegetables, for they engender a symphony of diversified nutrients conducive to overall vitality and metabolic equilibrium.

- Assimilation of Salubrious Lipids: The integration of sources of wholesome fats—avocado, nuts, seeds, olive oil, and fatty fish—commends itself. Such fats are integral to the bestowal of requisite nutrients and the harmonization of hormonal equanimity.

- The Praxis of Aromatics: Harness the potential of herbs and spices as vanguards of flavor enhancement sans recourse to surfeit salt or saccharine embellishment. Turmeric, cayenne, cinnamon, and ginger, among others, not only titillate palates but also confer metabolic invigoration.

- Complex Carbohydrate Incorporeality: Leverage the benefits of whole grains, an example of which is quinoa, brown rice, whole wheat pasta, and oats. The preponderance of these complex carbohydrates proffers sustained vitality and attendant fiber fortification.

Meticulous Gauging of Proportions: Exercising judiciousness in proportions is imperative. Subsuming superfluous quantities—even of nutrient-dense constituents—can inculcate counterproductive consequences.

Guidelines for Groceries:

- Anticipatory Predisposition: Anticipate the weekly alimentary regimen through the architectonics of a detailed meal stratagem before embarking upon grocery forays. This practice serves to circumvent superfluous acquisitions and undergirds prudent resource utilization.

- Strategic Sojourn through Perimeter: The circumambulation of the store's perimeter is of import. This domain typically enfolds an assortment of fresh produce, lean proteins, grains, and dairy—constituents quintessential to the Metabolic Confusion Diet.

- Cognizant Protein Elicitation: Embrace a diversification of lean protein selections, encompassing skinless poultry, lean meat avatars, piscine entities, tofu, and leguminous variants.

- Pallets Awash in Colorful Chromatics: Populate your cart with an expansive assortment of vegetables, be they fresh, frozen, or tinned sans superfluous sodium enhancements. A vivid vegetal tableau is indicative of nutritional profusion.

- Affirmation of Whole-Grain Dominion: Favour the election of whole grain envoys, such as whole wheat bread, quinoa, brown rice, and whole wheat pasta, that align cohesively with dietary dictums.

- Eminence of Sapid Lipid Mediums: Solicit the inclusion of nutrient-rich lipids—avocado, nuts, seeds, and olive oil—transcending culinary prerequisites to assume the role of metabolic agents.

- Herbal Embellishments: Assemble a diverse repertoire of spices conducive to metabolic stoking, wherein turmeric, cayenne pepper, and cinnamon hold sway.

- Refrain from Processed Comestibles: Eschew processed and saccharine-laden provisions, as their juxtaposition with the metabolic confusion ethos is incongruent.

- Label Scrutiny: When bespeaking packaged items, exercise circumspection in label perusal. Scrutiny thereof ensures the abeyance of undue sugars, deleterious fats, and egregious sodium augmentation.

- Hydration Overture: Inculcate hydration by procuring copious water and herbal infusions to accompany the dietary pilgrimage.

By assimilating these venerated cooking strategies and judicious grocery proclivities, confluence with the Metabolic Confusion Diet is attained whilst engendering sustenance profuse in nutrients. The confluence of constancy and equilibrium is the bedrock upon which the pinnacle of health and fitness aspirations are realized.

CHAPTER 8

LISTENING TO YOUR BODY: ADJUSTMENTS AND PLATEAUS

Recognizing Signs Your Body Gives You

Embarking on the journey of well-being necessitates an artful grasp of the messages your body conveys. Your body, an eloquent communicator, whispers its desires, reactions, and states through an array of cues. Let's delve into the realm of these cues, deciphering the intricate language of your body:

1. Hunger and Satisfaction:

Gentle Grumblings: That subtle rumble or playful gnawing in your stomach—your body's subtle plea for nourishment.

Satiety: The moment when contentment envelops you, marking the completion of a satisfying meal.

2. Energy Tides and Fatigue:

The Yawn of Lethargy: When fatigue envelops you like a warm blanket, signaling the need for rest or revitalization.

Sparkling Vitality: Feeling invigorated, wide-eyed, and ready to seize the day—an orchestra of energy harmonizing within.

3. The Whispers of Thirst:

Parched Whispers: A dry tongue or a gentle scratchiness—the body's gentle reminder to hydrate, to sip from life's wellspring.

The Call of Quenching: A thirst that beckons, urging you to heed the symphony of your body's fluid needs.

4. The Digestive Tango:

Bloat's Murmur: A discreet belly blooming, a puff of discomfort—your body's plea for a mindful rendezvous with digestion.

The Dance of Digestion: The ease of a well-danced tango, evidenced by comfort and regularity in your belly's movements.

5. Mood's Brushstrokes:

The Tempest Within: A storm of irritability brewing, clouds obscuring the sunshine—a signal for emotional recalibration.

The Sunlit Sky: A clear, tranquil emotional canvas, splashed with hues of serenity—a portrait of emotional equilibrium.

6. The Slumber Symphony:

The Insomniac's Tale: Tossing and turning, sleep's elusive embrace—a nocturnal sonnet hinting at unmet needs.

The Dreamer's Oasis: Awakening refreshed, dreams woven in the tapestry of slumber—a nocturnal rhapsody well-received.

7. Cravings' Symphony and Aversions' Lullaby:

Cravings' Crescendo: An orchestra of longing for particular tastes—a serenade of the body's subtle yearnings.

Aversions' Whispers: A gentle refrain of repulsion, a tug away from certain flavors—a body's discourse in culinary preferences.

8. Physical Echoes:

Headache's Echo: The drumbeat of discomfort, a pulsating rhythm hinting at the need for care and reprieve.

Muscle's Sonata: The melody of exertion, a harmonious reminder of your body's symphony in motion.

9. The Tapestry of Skin:

Skin's Whisper: The dry caress or blemished tales your skin tells—a mural of well-being painted in dermal hues.

Glowing Canvas: A canvas aglow, skin radiating health— an artistic portrayal of vitality etched on the body's parchment.

10. Heart's Beat and Breath's Sigh:

- Accelerated Rhythms: The racing heart, a pulse hastened—perhaps a melody of exertion or an echo of tension.

- Unison of Breath: The rise and fall of breath, a cadence in tranquil synchronization—a breath symphony in serene harmony.

11. The Inner Musings:

- The Foggy Chronicles: Thoughts shrouded in haze, a mental labyrinth—a gentle nudge for mindful engagement.

- Clarity's Anthem: Thoughts crystalline, a vista of mental clarity—a triumphant chorus of focused introspection.

12. Weight's Sonata: - Weight's Ebb and Flow: The scale's fluctuating melody—a rhythm charting the

cadence of lifestyle, offering a chapter in your body's book.

In embracing these signs, you embark on a journey of attuned mindfulness. Each cue, each murmur, weaves a narrative in your body's dialect. By heeding these whispers, you forge a harmonious partnership with your body's rhythm, choreographing a dance of wellness that echoes in the symphony of life.

Making Informed Adjustments to Your Approach

Embarking on any transformative journey, such as the Metabolic Confusion Diet, requires a dynamic approach that evolves alongside your changing needs and aspirations. Here, we unveil a comprehensive and strategic guide for making informed adjustments that not only align with your goals but also cater to the intricate interplay of your body and mind:

1. Consistent Self-Evaluation: Routinely set aside time to assess your progress and evaluate the effectiveness of your current approach.

Delve into the nuances of your achievements as well as areas that warrant attention and refinement.

Develop a heightened awareness of how your body responds to different stimuli, be it dietary changes or exercise routines.

2. Attuned Body Listening: Hone the art of tuning into your body's cues and signals, which often speak volumes about its needs.

Cultivate sensitivity to subtle shifts in energy levels, mood patterns, digestion, and overall well-being.

Grasp when your body communicates discomfort, fatigue, or the need for restorative interventions.

3. Data-Driven Progress Analysis: Harness quantitative metrics like changes in weight, body measurements, and fitness benchmarks.

Maintain meticulous records that serve as windows into the tapestry of your progress, enabling you to identify trends.

Enlist the guidance of health professionals to interpret these data points accurately and extract meaningful insights.

4. Seek Expert Input: Engage with professionals versed in nutrition, fitness, or medical expertise aligned with your chosen path.

Leverage their specialized knowledge to decipher progress and formulate nuanced adjustments.

By incorporating their insights, you can ensure that your adjustments are grounded in informed guidance.

5. Gradual Refinements: Introduce modifications to your approach gradually, avoiding abrupt shifts that could disrupt your equilibrium.

Observe meticulously how your body reacts to each modification, allowing for an accurate assessment of its impact.

The gradual approach facilitates a more precise understanding of cause-and-effect dynamics.

6. Delve into Nutritional Insights: Record your daily dietary intake through a food journal or digital apps for comprehensive tracking.

Analyze the distribution of macronutrients—carbohydrates, proteins, fats—to align with your body's unique requirements.

Based on your goals, adjust portion sizes, ratios, and meal timing for optimal nourishment.

7. Embrace Culinary Diversity: Infuse variety into your diet and exercise routines to prevent plateaus and sustain engagement.

Experiment with novel recipes, explore different workout modalities and introduce diverse nutrient sources.

This diversity not only fosters physical progress but also keeps your enthusiasm and motivation ignited.

8. Prioritize Recovery and Rest: Dedicate attention to your body's recovery needs, allowing ample time for recuperation between intense workouts.

Monitor the quality and duration of your sleep, and tailor your schedule to ensure optimal rejuvenation.

Recognize that optimal progress is underpinned by adequate recovery and well-being.

9. Flexibility for Adaptation: Cultivate flexibility within your routines to accommodate variations in energy levels, daily commitments, and unforeseen events.

Adapting gracefully to different contexts prevents disruptions and empowers seamless integration of your approach.

10. Periodic Reflective Assessment: Set intervals for comprehensive assessments of your evolving strategy to ascertain its efficacy.

- Scrutinize whether your adjustments yield the intended outcomes and pinpoint areas for further refinement.

- This cyclical process of reflection ensures that your approach remains aligned with your evolving journey.

11. Psychological Equilibrium: Acknowledge the profound impact of your journey on your psychological well-being.

- Be attuned to stressors, emotional responses, and mental resilience, recognizing the interconnectedness of body and mind.

- Adjustments should encompass strategies that foster a harmonious balance between physical progress and emotional health.

12. Perpetual Learning and Growth: Cultivate an attitude of continuous learning by staying updated on evolving research, trends, and holistic practices.

- Engage in workshops, read reputable sources, and participate in communities to deepen your knowledge base.

- This commitment to education ensures that your adjustments are well-informed and aligned with the latest insights.

Dealing with Plateaus: Strategies to Break Through

Conquering plateaus, those stubborn stages of stagnant progress require finesse and strategy on your path to optimal well-being. Here, we unveil a toolkit of savvy approaches to shatter plateaus and usher in revitalized progress, inching you closer to your goals:

1. In-Depth Analysis and Adjustment:

Holistic Scrutiny: Delve deep into your current routine, encompassing diet, exercise, and lifestyle choices.

Spotting Stagnation: Identify the points where progress has slowed down or become static.

Customized Tweaks: Tailor your adjustments to specifically target the areas showing signs of stagnation.

2. Rethinking Your Regimen:

Spice Up Workouts: Infuse variety by tweaking your workout routines to challenge diverse muscle groups and energy systems.

Intensity and Duration: Play with the intensity, duration, and frequency of your workouts to invigorate adaptation.

Unleash Novelty: Explore new exercises, classes, or sports to reignite the spark of excitement.

3. Reevaluating Nutrition:

Calorie Manipulation: Tune your caloric intake to match your evolving goals and energy expenditure.

Macro Mastery: Adjust macronutrient ratios to align with your body's evolving demands.

Micro Boost: Ensure you're nourishing your body with essential micronutrients for peak performance.

4. Power of Progressive Overload:

Scaling Weights: Gradually raise weights, resistance, or intensity to continuously challenge your muscles.

Elevating Endurance: Extend the duration or intensity of your cardio sessions progressively.

Skill Amplification: Elevate your competence and proficiency within your chosen activities.

5. Embrace Periodization:

Structured Phases: Segment your training into distinct phases, each with its unique goals and intensities.

Cyclic Mastery: Alternate between high-intensity, low-volume phases, and vice versa.

Adaptation Prevention: Keep your body guessing and growing by cycling through varied stimuli.

6. Prioritizing Recovery:

Rest and Rejuvenation: Give sleep, rest days, and relaxation the priority they deserve for optimal recovery.

Active Recharge: Include lighter activities like yoga or gentle stretches to aid in active recovery.

7. Mind-Muscle Connection:

Mindful Engagement: Channel laser-like focus onto the muscles you're targeting during strength training.

Form Finesse: Emphasize precise form and controlled movements over mere weight lifting.

8. Taming Stress:

Stress-Busting: Incorporate stress-relieving techniques such as meditation, deep breathing, or mindfulness.

Cortisol Control: Manage cortisol levels as persistently high cortisol can hinder progress.

9. Strength in Community:

Accountability Allies: Share your goals with a friend or join a community to stay on track.

Shared Journeys: Connecting with others facing similar challenges can provide encouragement and insights.

10. Mental Fortitude:

- Resilience and Perseverance: Understand that plateaus are a natural part of any journey.

- Positive Mindset: Foster a growth mindset, seeing obstacles as stepping stones to growth.

11. Professional Guidance:

- Expert Consultation: Seek advice from seasoned trainers, nutritionists, or healthcare professionals.

- Fresh Perspectives: Professionals can provide valuable insights and tailored strategies.

12. Goal Refinement:

- Reassessing Ambitions: Consider if your goals need fine-tuning based on your progress.

- Celebrating Victories: Recognize small wins along the way, bolstering your motivation.

CHAPTER 9

SUSTAINABLE LIFESTYLE HABITS BEYOND THE DIET

In the grand tapestry of well-being, dietary choices are merely a thread interwoven with numerous other elements that contribute to your overall vitality. Embracing sustainable health goes beyond the confines of what's on your plate, encompassing a symphony of practices that harmonize with your body, mind, and soul. Let's embark on a comprehensive exploration of these multifaceted lifestyle habits that extend far beyond the boundaries of diet:

1. Mindful Movement:

Diverse Physical Engagement: Regularly participate in activities that resonate with your preferences, be it invigorating runs, tranquil yoga sessions, dance classes, or team sports.

Consistency with Compassion: Prioritize consistent movement over sporadic bursts of intensity, fostering a lifelong relationship with physical activity.

Embrace Holistic Fitness: Combine cardiovascular exercises for heart health with strength training to enhance muscle integrity and overall resilience.

2. Quality Sleep:

Structured Sleep Routines: Establish a predictable sleep schedule, ensuring you attain 7-9 hours of rejuvenating rest each night.

Sleep Sanctuary: Craft an environment conducive to sleep by minimizing external disruptions such as noise and light.

Pre-Sleep Rituals: Develop calming bedtime rituals, such as reading a book or practicing meditation, to prepare your mind for rest.

3. Mastery of Stress:

Stress-Alleviating Techniques: Regularly engage in practices like deep breathing, meditation, or mindfulness to counteract the effects of stress.

Joy-Fueled Pursuits: Cultivate hobbies and activities that resonate with your passions, offering a therapeutic outlet for stress release.

Mindful Work-Life Balance: Strive for equilibrium between work and personal life, guarding against chronic stress and fostering overall well-being.

4. Hydration Rituals:

Hydrate Mindfully: Prioritize consistent water intake throughout the day to support bodily functions and maintain hydration.

Expanded Beverage Repertoire: Infuse variety into hydration by incorporating herbal teas and water infusions for a burst of flavor and additional benefits.

Heed Body Signals: Tune into your body's thirst cues and respond promptly to maintain optimal hydration levels.

5. Nurturing Relationships:

Connection Nurtures Well-being: Dedicate time to nurturing meaningful relationships, investing in shared experiences and open communication.

Active Listening and Empathy: Foster emotional connections by practicing active listening and demonstrating empathy in interactions.

Social Support as Pillar: Recognize that strong social networks contribute to emotional well-being, resilience, and a sense of belonging.

6. Mindful Eating:

Attuned Nourishment: Cultivate mindful eating by tuning into hunger and satiety cues, savoring each bite, and appreciating the sensory experience.

Whole-Food Choices: Opt for nutrient-dense, whole foods that nourish your body and provide sustained energy throughout the day.

Unplugged Eating: Minimize distractions during meals, allowing yourself to fully engage with and enjoy your food.

7. Personal Flourishing:

Goal-Setting with Purpose: Define personal and professional goals that align with your passions, values, and vision of growth.

Lifelong Learning: Foster a spirit of curiosity by consistently pursuing learning opportunities through reading, workshops, or online courses.

Reflective Progression: Periodically reflect on your journey, celebrate achievements, and recalibrate goals in alignment with your evolving self.

8. Nourishing Mental Health: Holistic Self-Care: Prioritize self-care activities that resonate with your well-

being, whether it's spending time in nature, engaging in hobbies, or practicing mindfulness.

Professional Guidance: Seek professional help when needed to address mental health concerns and develop effective coping mechanisms.

Empowering Self-Image: Cultivate a positive self-image, practicing self-compassion and embracing your uniqueness.

9. Digital Detox Retreats:

Balanced Screen Time: Establish boundaries around screen usage, designating tech-free periods during meals and before bedtime.

Presence in the Moment: Immerse yourself in activities that cultivate present-moment awareness, such as meditation, nature walks, or creative pursuits.

Rekindle Real Connections: Disconnecting from screens fosters genuine connections with yourself, others, and the world around you.

10. Mindful Environmental Stewardship: - Eco-Conscious Practices: Reduce your ecological footprint by embracing eco-friendly choices like recycling, composting, and using reusable items.

- Sustainable Mobility: Opt for planet-friendly transportation modes, like walking, cycling, or utilizing public transit.

- Supporting Local and Organic: Prioritize local and organic products to contribute to a healthier planet and a more sustainable future.

11. Gratitude and Positive Resonance:

- Daily Gratitude Practice: Dedicate moments to express gratitude for the positives in your life, fostering a sense of contentment and abundance.

- Constructive Optimism: Cultivate a positive outlook by focusing on solutions rather than dwelling on challenges.

- Surroundings and Affirmations: Create an environment that bolsters positivity through inspiring surroundings and uplifting affirmations.

12. Leisurely Rejuvenation: - Holistic Leisure: Carve out time for leisure activities that bring joy, relaxation, and a sense of rejuvenation.

- Nurturing Hobbies: Engage in hobbies and creative pursuits that fuel your passion, stimulate creativity, and offer an outlet for self-expression.

- Balancing Act: Balancing work commitments with leisure pursuits contributes to overall life satisfaction and a harmonious lifestyle.

By weaving this rich tapestry of lifestyle habits into the fabric of your daily existence, you create a multi-dimensional symphony of well-being that extends well beyond dietary considerations. Embracing this holistic approach nurtures not only your physical health but also enriches your mental, emotional, social, and spiritual dimensions. Remember, sustainable wellness is an ongoing journey, a reflection of mindful choices and intentional living that manifests in a life brimming with vitality and meaning.

CONCLUSION

As we conclude our exploration into the Metabolic Confusion Diet for endomorph women and the broader realm of sustainable health, it's clear that the pursuit of well-being is a dynamic and intricate journey. Our voyage has spanned body types, metabolic strategies, hormonal intricacies, nutrition, fitness, mental wellness, and lifestyle habits, revealing a holistic tapestry that extends far beyond mere dietary considerations.

Our journey commenced by understanding the distinct landscapes of body types - ectomorphs, mesomorphs, and endomorphs - where genetics shape our responses to nutrition and exercise. For endomorph women, the Metabolic Confusion Diet emerges as a bespoke approach, harnessing caloric variation, macronutrient cycling, and intermittent fasting to optimize metabolism and ignite progress.

Delving into the world of endomorph characteristics, challenges, and strengths, we've underscored the importance of embracing individuality and forging a partnership with our bodies. Unpacking the intricate dance between hormones and metabolic rates emphasized the pivotal role of hormonal equilibrium in holistic well-being.

Navigating through macronutrient cycling, caloric variations, and their harmony with intermittent fasting, we've illuminated the art of sustaining metabolic dynamism and transcending plateaus. Coupled with tailored workout strategies, including invigorating cardiovascular exercise, these methods paint a vivid picture of a holistic fitness journey.

Beyond the physical, we've embarked on a journey of psychological well-being, confronting cravings, navigating social landscapes, and charting progress. Recognizing meal prepping's role in sustained success, we've equipped ourselves with the tools to make conscious choices even amidst life's hustle.

Through quick, nutrient-dense recipes, we've savored the joys of culinary creation, linking nutritional nourishment with the broader mosaic of well-being. Moreover, our narrative has traversed grocery aisles, decoded bodily cues, explored informed adaptations, and embraced a balanced lifestyle that resonates profoundly.

This voyage has cultivated not just insights, but also a sense of empowerment. Empowered with knowledge, strategies, and a panoramic view, you're poised to navigate the ever-evolving seas of well-being with a confident stride. Remember, this journey is exclusively yours - a canvas awaiting the brushstrokes of your choices, the hues of your aspirations, and the masterpiece of your flourishing.

As you step forward from these pages, may you embark on a lifelong odyssey of self-discovery, growth, and nurturing. Beyond dietary boundaries, you're summoned to embrace a life where diet, exercise, mindfulness, relationships, and personal evolution harmonize into a symphony of vibrant well-being.

With each chapter you pen, each adaptation you craft, and every milestone you celebrate, you embody the architect of a narrative that is uniquely yours - a story destined to be both extraordinary and fulfilling.

Printed in Great Britain
by Amazon

41291922R00086